Praise for *A Good Birth*

"Groundbreaking. . . . Reading this book brings you back to your own birth stories and will change the way you not only feel about them but also the way you discuss and share them. In other words, it's a must-read for every mother."

—AllParenting.com

"The book is laced with heartfelt anecdotes and compelling stories from new mothers. . . . Acknowledging the pros and cons of both sides of the debates, Lyerly writes with candor and humility."

—*The Boston Globe*

"Lyerly aims to make doctors, moms, and moms-to-be feel less judgmental about other people's choices and more empowered when it comes to their own."

—*Booklist*

"Directly yet compassionately addresses the issues surrounding what constitutes an unconstrained 'good' birth and the primary goals associated with it. . . . [Lyerly's] comforting and informational guidebook will be useful for those seeking to explore the less-obvious components of parturition. Positive, sympathetic and diverse perspectives for past, present and future mothers-to-be."

—*Kirkus Reviews*

"Insightful . . . [Lyerly] has an important message."   —*Publishers Weekly*

"Dr. Lyerly has cut through the noise of the 'birth wars' to let women's voices ring through. Maternity care providers, whether they subscribe to medical or midwifery models, should listen. This book is a gift to women who have or will ever give birth."

—Lisa Harris, M.D., Ph.D., Department of Obstetrics and Gynecology and Department of Women's Studies, University of Michigan

"In listening to women, Lyerly has done much more than give them a voice; she has distilled women's hopes and fears, their passions, their love and their wisdom into a transformative vision of what birth means for all of us. This inspiring book restores women to the center of birth and makes crystal-clear what women have always known to be true: birth matters, deeply, widely, and lastingly."

—Elizabeth Mitchell Armstrong, Associate Professor, Sociology and Public Affairs, Princeton University

"Dr. Lyerly represents the new generation of women obstetrician-gynecologists who bring a new sensitivity and appreciation to what has also been a gendered debate, since male physicians hitherto predominated in the specialty. She pursues a reassessment of the intersection of medicine and culture, authority and autonomy, professionalism and patients. This book will inform all who care that women should truly experience the 'best birth possible.'"

—Timothy R.B. Johnson M.D., FACOG, Bates Professor of the Diseases of Women and Children, and Chair, Department of Obstetrics and Gynecology Professor of Women's Studies, University of Michigan

"Lyerly skillfully and sensitively helps prospective mothers identify what matters most to them as they enter the increasingly complex world of maternity care options, underscoring the importance of collaboration amongst all caregivers to better support women."

—Judy Norsigian, Executive Director, Our Bodies Ourselves

"*A Good Birth* is like no other book in the pregnancy and birthing literature. Annie Lyerly's beautiful prose helps all of us understand what we each should do, and expect of one another, to make every birth a good birth."

—Ruth R. Faden, Ph.D., MPH, Philip Franklin Wagley Professor of Biomedical Ethics and Director, Johns Hopkins Berman Institute of Bioethics

"*A Good Birth* radically repositions our understanding of what makes childbirth valuable and meaningful to women. Dr. Anne Lyerly adds a crucial perspective to our understanding of birth, full of rich insights based on the experiences of women themselves."

—Elena Gates, M.D., Professor, Department of Obstetrics, Gynecology and Reproductive Sciences, University of California, San Francisco

"What *Dying Well* did to revolutionize caring practices around dying, this book does for caring practices around giving birth. Mandatory reading for health practitioners and policy makers."

—Margaret Olivia Little, Ph.D., Director, Kennedy Institute for Ethics and Associate Professor of Philosophy, Georgetown University

A Good Birth

Finding the Positive and Profound in Your Childbirth Experience

Anne Drapkin Lyerly, M.D.

AVERY

A member of Penguin Group (USA)

New York

AVERY

Published by the Penguin Group
Penguin Group (USA) LLC
375 Hudson Street
New York, New York 10014

USA · Canada · UK · Ireland · Australia
New Zealand · India · South Africa · China

penguin.com
A Penguin Random House Company

First trade paperback edition 2014
Copyright © 2013 by Anne Lyerly

Most Avery books are available at special quantity discounts for bulk purchase for sales promotions, premiums, fund-raising, and educational needs. Special books or book excerpts also can be created to fit specific needs. For details, write Special .Markets@us.penguingroup.com.

The Library of Congress has catalogued the hardcover edition as follows:

Lyerly, Anne Drapkin.
    A good birth : finding the positive and profound in your childbirth experience / Anne Drapkin Lyerly, M.D.
        p.   cm.
Includes bibliographical references and index.
    ISBN 978-1-58333-498-0
1. Childbirth—Case studies.   2. Childbirth—Psychological aspects—Case studies.   3. Pregnancy—
Psychological aspects—Case studies.   I. Title.
    RG658.L94   2013
    618.2—dc23   2013015206

ISBN 978-1-58333-549-9 (paperback)

Printed in the United States of America
10 9 8 7 6 5 4 3 2 1

BOOK DESIGN BY MICHELLE MCMILLIAN

To my mom and dad,
Nancy and Paul Drapkin

To Kim and our sweet brood,
Grant, Paul, Charlie, Will, and Grace

With unending love and gratitude

Contents

A
Good
Birth

In Search of a Good Birth

Only when the conscious experience of mothers, potential mothers, and mothering persons are taken fully into account can we possibly develop understanding that might someday merit the description of "human."

—VIRGINIA HELD

It is important to remember that the writers [of the history of childbirth] were by no means disinterested, that they were engaged in both a rhetorical and political battle—and that the one group whose opinions and documentation we long to have—the mothers—are, as usual, almost entirely unheard from.

—ADRIENNE RICH

"This belonged to your grandmother," my mom said as she placed the soup tureen on the kitchen counter. It bore the patina of age and was modest in size, adorned with rosebuds, reflective of both the restraint (or the dearth) and craftsmanship that characterized the time.

Grant, the oldest of my four boys, was just a few weeks old and we were visiting my mom in Palo Alto. She and I weren't planning on cooking—our evenings together now invariably meant plated takeout by candlelight whenever the baby would allow.

Indeed, there was more to the tureen than met the eye. It was not just a container for soup—far from it. Rather, my mom told me, it is where I was bathed in my first weeks of life. It was hard to imagine. She slipped her hands inside it, cupping them as if holding a tiny infant. I was full-term, but a peanut by all accounts, and apparently fit just fine in the diminutive container.

Maybe she just wanted to show it to me, but her digging it out was no small feat, and my sense has always been that she wanted to communicate something more. One possibility is that it was a confession—yes, I was small, and somehow that was her "fault"—something that carried an element of shame for her, despite the fact that 1960s obstetricians counseled their patients to limit weight gain to ten or fifteen pounds, and allowed for (even encouraged) smoking if it helped in the effort to remain svelte. My mom—a peanut herself when she emerged from the hospital with me—somehow dutifully managed to follow her doctor's burdensome and unfounded advice.

But I think the tureen was about something else. I think it was an effort, however subtle, to put a little salve on the wound that was my cesarean. No doubt I felt guilty about it, inadequate for it, confused by my inability to deliver the "right" or "normal" way. It was nothing like my own birth—quick, vaginal, and remembered and recounted with great fondness by both my parents. But if my mom had a euphoric experience, she wanted to remind me, she did it in the context of pushing out a baby half Grant's size.

The tureen was exactly what I needed. My husband (bless his heart) had gotten nowhere with me in his efforts to attribute my delivery mode to the fact that Grant's head circumference was in the ninety-ninth percentile. But the tureen and my mother communicated what I needed to hear—that it was all right, that I had nothing to be ashamed of, that I'd given birth beautifully to a beautiful boy.

I've often wished I could pull out a tureen—for patients and friends, even strangers in whose eyes I see a semblance of regret. I suppose that is, in large part, what this book is about. It's about crafting a notion of the good that doesn't turn on time or place or event, in which shame and regret haven't a place, in which births can be celebrated for all the ways that they are utterly worthy of our deepest regard.

In Search of a Good Birth

The encounter with my grandmother's soup tureen marked the beginning of a decade's effort on my part to understand how women think about their births, why they think about them as they do, and what it is that I might have to offer—as a mother, doctor, and researcher—to broad debates about the state of maternity care in the United States and worldwide.

Most of us agree that something is amiss. The rate of cesareans is higher than it should be; in the United States, we spend more on birth and have worse outcomes than scores of other industrialized nations; women's choices about birth remain inexplicably and irrationally constrained. You have heard all these things, I am sure. What you have not heard but perhaps know all too well—from experiencing birth or talking to those who have—is that even when mom and baby are healthy, giving birth often leaves women looking back on the event with some degree of uncertainty or sadness. They ask what happened, whether it was justified, and perhaps most pointedly how it reflects on them as mothers, women, people. Even women who have come to celebrate their experience either find themselves defending their choices, insisting they shouldn't have to, or providing comfort or context to those for whom uncertainty or regret colors the day.

Having worked on issues related to birth for the past twenty years, I've come to believe that the heart of the problem is not just with the "system" or with certain types of practitioners or approaches to birth. The heart of the problem is a deep confusion about the goals of birth—about what it is that makes a birth "good."

What makes for a good birth? That emerged for me as *the* pressing question as I watched a cavalcade of doctors, midwives, celebrities, and talking heads appear in the media, bicker on blogs, and advocate for a wide variety of different birthing practices. From the American College of Obstetricians and Gynecologists' position against home birth to talk-show host Ricki Lake's film and book about the virtues of "natural" delivery, it seems everyone has an opinion—and an agenda.

Read any book on the issue and you will sense a bias, either toward the notion that birth is normal and natural and not the proper place for medicine, or toward the notion that birth is complicated, potentially risky, and responsibly undertaken only in the context of medical care, in a hospital. These two views of birth are often respectively ascribed to the professions that most frequently espouse them—the midwifery view on one side and the medical view on the other, while some have marked these approaches with different words, like *holistic* and *technocratic*.

These views mark the edges of a polarized debate over where birth should be undertaken and how, who is the presumptive attendant, which professionals need to be supervised, and which way the money should flow—what I'll refer to throughout the book as the "birth wars." At the heart of each view is a very different idea of what we're after in birth—what it is that makes a birth *good*. Beyond the sheer unpleasantness of the bickering, the fact is that neither side has it quite right, and together these divergent views of the good birth leave childbearing women wondering whom to believe in anticipation of birth, and what went wrong once it has happened.

This book is an effort to redress this state of affairs by giving voice to women themselves—women who've been through birth, who've had a chance to think about what really matters in the process of bringing a child into the world. It is an effort to craft a notion of the good birth that turns not on the concrete things about which doctors and midwives tussle, but on what women say is deeply at issue for them.

But before I turn to mothers, let's take a look at the two views that dominate conversations about birth, the reasons why neither one has it quite right, and the damage they both inflict in the process.

Two Views of Birth

To look at the medical literature, you'd think that there is just one measure of a good birth: the health of mom and baby. When medicine assesses how it's doing, we look at what are often called "discrete medical outcomes." Some of these are familiar to those who have been through it: a baby's weight at birth, the Apgar score (a quick assessment done on all babies one and five minutes post-birth, which gives a sense of how their transition into the world is going, how healthy and vigorous they appear, and whether they might need medical assistance), gestational age (how close to the due date a baby is born), and a range of maternal complications, such as how much blood a mom loses or whether and how much she tears, to name a few.

Of course these issues are critically important. Trends in a breadth of discrete medical outcomes reflect the quality of care childbearing women and babies alike receive. But just as surely, a good medical outcome and a good birth, while sometimes concomitant, are not one and the same.

Take for instance the tale of Elizabeth Rourke, spun elegantly by surgeon and writer Atul Gawande in a 2006 *New Yorker* essay titled "The Score." Elizabeth, an internal medicine doctor and recent mother, spoke to Gawande about what she had hoped her birth would be like—hopes shared (in one form or another) by a generous proportion of first-time mothers in contemporary America: "I wanted no intervention, no doctors, no drugs," she said. "In a perfect world, I wanted to have my baby in a forest bower attended by fairy sprites." Instead, she ended up with a long hospital labor, an epidural, a cesarean, and, in her words, a "totally gorgeous little child" with a nearly perfect Apgar score. For medicine, the birth was no doubt a success. But Elizabeth, according to Gawande, was a self-proclaimed "wreck." And it wasn't the cesarean scar she was talking about. It was, instead, a complete sense of failure in the aftermath of a birth that didn't go as she had hoped.

Or Elise, a mom I met a couple of years ago at a local park: As we watched her son, who was sandwiched in age (and literally at times) between my now two sons Grant and Paul, our small talk turned to what we did for a living. She had been working at a bioresearch company as a project manager for the past five years. I told her about my career in obstetrics and my recent research project that involved interviewing mothers about what they considered a good birth (The Good Birth Project—more about this soon).

Elise needed no prompting to tell me about her own birthing experience and the trauma she experienced in its midst. She was at the hospital in active labor when her baby's heart rate dropped precipitously. The staff put an oxygen mask on her face and asked her to turn over, from back to front, to shift her weight and the baby's to improve the flow of oxygen through the umbilical cord.

"So there I was," she continued, "on my hands and knees, someone holding an oxygen mask to my face, another person with their hand in my vagina. Tears were streaming down my face—I was terrified.

"And then the nurse asked me . . ." She paused, biting her lip to keep from tearing up. "'Honey, why are you crying?'"

Elise gestured at her rambunctious five-year-old, busy talking trucks with my sons. "My baby is healthy and gorgeous, but that nurse's comment is the thing that keeps coming back to me when I think about the day he was born."

Elise's story echoes a point that so many women know or come to understand: a good medical outcome doesn't necessarily make for a good birth. Yet that's what was emphasized to me in medical school—as a doctor, as long as you follow medical procedures and as long as the mom and baby go home healthy, you have done your job. The medical literature focuses nearly exclusively on health outcomes, narrowly construed. We know there's more to it, but what exactly?

If you turn to the other side of the birthing argument, you'll find that advocates of natural childbirth and midwifery have offered answers; but their answers, if full of wisdom in many ways, bring problems of their own. According to the so-called midwifery view, it is not just medicine's approach to birth, but its use of and reliance on technology that is at the root of modern women's dissatisfaction. People on that side of the birth debate often equate a good birth with a "natural" or "normal" event, free of drugs and medical interventions, often in a more personal setting than a hospital delivery room.

It's a view I came to appreciate at the end of my training in obstetrics, and I will say that, at first glance, it intrigued me. Much of what I read resonated for me in the aftermath of the physically, emotionally—and morally—grueling process of residency. In learning medicine's approach to pregnancy and birth, I often didn't like what I saw and what I was told to do—indeed, sometimes what I did—in delivery rooms. I worried about my patients and what they took away (besides a baby) from their experience on the maternity ward. I appreciated midwifery's emphasis on the importance of the connectedness between the woman and her baby—not two separate patients, but a "unit" whose interests often aligned, whose well-being was intimately intertwined. I agreed with the emphasis on "woman-centeredness" and on the importance of crafting the birth experience around the things that mattered most to women. I loved that they emphasized that birth is more than a biological event—that it has enduring meaning for women, families, and society.

What I didn't find convincing, though, was the way that obstetrics' critics held medicine and, more pointedly, *technology* as centrally culpable for what was wrong with maternity care; the ways they linked, and closely, absence of technology with the "good"; the view that Elizabeth Rourke's (the new mom from Gawande's tale) version of the low-intervention birth is the way to go: that in birth, medicine is largely misplaced.

If you think this is too stark a characterization, consider the "Optimality Index" that has been proposed as a measure of maternity care quality and endorsed by the American College of Nurse-Midwives. Its advocates point to the fact that it "shifts the measurement focus from adverse to good outcomes, and counts the frequency of 'optimal' events during childbirth." Good so far. The problem is in how *optimal* is defined—it is the "lack of interventions during a woman's perinatal experience." So a required medication, a desired epidural, and even a lifesaving blood transfusion reduce your score. If the midwifery community wants to measure and mark the level of medical intervention in birth, fine. But the term *optimality* implies that less intervention is necessarily better, that a good birth is by definition low intervention. But for many women, this is far from the case.

Indeed, in birth, less is not always more. I have been around birth long enough to know that a birth's "naturalness" (or what some advocates call "normalcy") is as misleading a metric of the "good" as is medical outcome. Not everyone wants a "natural" birth—some women find comfort in ready access to technology and reasonably desire things like pain medicine. Further, the emphasis on low-tech births has the potential to contribute to unhappy and sometimes traumatic experiences when physiology and circumstance, the unknowns of birth that can arise in the most uncomplicated pregnancies, make medical intervention prudent, necessary, even lifesaving. And for women who do not have access to such "normal births" by virtue of their health needs, personal needs, or limited access to birthing options—this notion of the good birth alienates or confuses those who may already have drawn a short straw in the lottery of life, reproductive or otherwise.

Certainly, modern medicine has overreached—doctors have harmed women (and men) with the misuse of technology. I am as aware as anyone of the well-worn examples from the obstetrics of prior decades: the use of heavy anesthesia to induce "twilight sleep" and other forms of maternal detachment; the "prophylactic" use of episiotomy and forceps for all birthing women; shaving, enemas, and the like. During my residency, I'd worked with (and had been trained by) doctors who had practiced during those darker times, and their contemporary practice showed echoes of the problematic past. And further, I had heard about such offenses firsthand from my mother: unmedicated and on the brink of delivering my older brother in Washington, D.C.'s posh Sibley Hospital in 1967, she was—apparently per protocol, as historians note was common at the time—knocked out and her baby was pulled from her with forceps. Decades after, my otherwise equanimous father would recall with a shudder the number of needle sticks in my mother's back, the purple mark that graced my brother's brow for days after his birth, and the feelings of violation that remained for many years after the bodily scars on his wife and child had healed.

No doubt there is something terribly wrong about the injudicious use of technology in the context of birth, which remains widespread if in somewhat less blatant forms (the unreflective use of external fetal monitoring for uncomplicated births, as an example, has led to more cesarean deliveries but no fewer cases of cerebral palsy, and comes at the cost of immobilizing birthing women who want and need mobility). But it doesn't follow that the use of technology in all circumstances should be construed negatively; and perhaps more to the point, it doesn't follow that a birth *without* technology is thereby a good one.

For one, if such were true, many women would simply be left out. Women, for example, whose health conditions require medical intervention to usher them safely through—the woman with a heart condition that precludes her safely pushing a child from her body, for whom the use of epidural and forceps *allow* a safe vaginal birth; or the woman with a uterine scar for whom contractions carry a considerable chance of uterine rupture and its potentially catastrophic risks, including death of the childbearing woman and her baby. No doubt, when forced upon a woman giving birth, anesthesia, forceps, or cesarean can be deeply harmful—violating. But it remains true that their respectful and judicious use can be welcome, helpful, and sometimes lifesaving. It seemed unlikely and unfair to me that some women's physiological misfortune should mean that a birth that was both "good" and safe was beyond their reach. But what might the good entail when technology was needed or desired?

A better answer might have helped my friend Erin sort out her feelings about her recent birth experience—which left her with a healthy baby as well as a hefty portion of what she termed "mama guilt about needing intervention." She'd planned and hoped for a home birth, but after forty-eight hours of labor at home, was transferred to the hospital, and ultimately delivered vaginally in the operating room.

"It was a far cry from the candlelit room in the birthing tub where I'd started pushing," she told me, "but incredible and wonderful too. We got a goddess OB who made the OR feel as home-birthy as possible. Our midwife and doula were present and involved. Mike caught the baby."

In the end—and in the midst of guilt about a birth that didn't go as planned—she called the experience "perfect." But it wasn't what she hoped for—wasn't "optimal" according to the version of birthing she'd embraced.

You might think that Erin was confused or wishful, or just plain unable in such close proximity to the event to call the birth of the child she adored anything but perfect. But I think something else was going on. I think Erin had a "good birth" that just didn't line up with anything she'd ever read about; it didn't line up with her preconceived (and understandably so) notion of what makes for good births—a notion marked by homelike settings and candlelit tubs.

And so Erin and many others emerge with "mama guilt." Its source, I'm convinced, is a distorted notion of the good birth that is rooted in professional agendas rather than the perspectives and experiences of women themselves. For many of us, the birth of a child is among life's most memorable and emotional experiences. That those memories are imbued with regret or uncertainty because of the way our culture talks and thinks about birth—the way doctors and midwives and women themselves squabble about it—is something I'm determined to change.

Women who have given birth, and have had time to think about it, pull away from entrenched mantras—they can tell you, and have told me, what made their births good. When I started looking and listening, I heard whispers of the things that mattered deeply to women. At first, they made their way to me through poetry and literature; slipped through lines of books advocating one mantra or the other; emerged in the hundreds of responses often mounted to contemporary articles about birth; and came through historical accounts of birth, particularly when women's voices were used as primary sources. Once I started listening, I became convinced that there was a different way of looking at and talking about birth—that women were doing this already, but their voices were buried in the din of what has been for the most part a professional and political debate.

There is another piece to this situation, another piece to my certainty that what is missing is a nuanced and woman-centered view of the good birth. For the misunderstandings around birth have a powerful analogue at the other bookend of life. Indeed, the question "What is a good death?" has animated scholarly work and public debate for at least the past two decades. If modern medicine has a complicated relationship with birth, its relationship with death is far from simple. In his book *Dying Well*, palliative care doctor Ira Byock reflected on the absence, during his early years as a physician, of the "good death from discussions in the medical and pastoral literature and at conferences." He added, "Without a consistent language and conceptual model for the range of human experiences at life's end, a taxonomy to label what we clinically saw, it was as if the phenomena did not actually exist."

Some people I know and love say that's true, that there is no such thing as a good death, that death defies what we can consider a source of good, that it is a deep sea of meaninglessness. But my experience has suggested otherwise. A year before my encounter with the soup tureen, my father died— unexpectedly, tragically, and I daresay well. If that day and those that followed were full of sorrow, we all were also grateful for a certain sweetness the process of his death imparted. For all of us who were there to experience it, the *way* he died has been a source of solace. We gathered at his bedside, held his hands, told stories, wiped his tears and our own. He held on after he was disconnected from the ventilator, continued along in the sacred space we'd crafted in the intensive care unit, then seemed to go when he was ready, when only the people he loved most were there, crossing his hands together as he took his last breath. His was a gentle, respectful departure—that no doubt has carried me through dark days since, and buoyed me in the lighter ones as well.

Medicine has learned some hard lessons about the end of life over the past several decades—not the least of which is that death is not just the enemy. *How* death happens, not just that it does, matters. It shapes the way we think about the people we have lost; it shapes the way we imagine our own lives.

In recent years, considerable effort has been made to understand what matters at the end of life and to pull it into reach. Many researchers have looked to dying patients to understand what we might do to helpfully shape their final weeks and days. Theorists have worked to understand why we behave the way we do around death. Policy makers have worked to help people get access to things like palliative care. Interestingly enough, many of those focused on death have put childbirth on a pedestal and have said that dying should be more like giving birth—it should be an opportunity for joy and meaning. As Byock put it, "When the human dimension of dying is nurtured, for many the transition from life can become as profound, intimate and precious as the miracle of birth."

I wish birth actually earned that sort of keep, but all too often it doesn't. I am afraid that we in obstetrics are similarly shortsighted when it comes to the bookend of life we most frequently attend. If we were appalled in the mid-1990s at figures that indicated that most Americans die alone, in pain, and not according to their wishes—the fact that that might be happening also at the beginning of life has evaded too many of us. Much of the time, birth as idealized turns out to be a far cry from the messy and complicated truth that the making of mothers, fathers, and children turns out to be.

With my father's death, I started reading and thinking about death with a sort of urgency. I was struck by questions that rang familiar: What is the role of pain and pain control in facilitating a good death? Where is the "right" place to die? At home, in a hospital, in a freestanding facility? Does technology undermine or facilitate a "good death," and in what ways? Insert *birth* in place of *death* and there you have the contemporary debate about birth in America. But the most pressing similarity, it occurred to me, was this inattention, this unwillingness to listen, to understand what mattered most to the people going through it. Much progress has been made concerning what it is that patients and families understand makes for a good death. Among the wisdom reaped from studying experiences at the end of life is that the goal is not an idealized or scripted death, but a death that aims at participating in certain goods, like the ones I experienced at my father's bedside. It seemed well past time for a similar inquiry around life's beginning.

And so began the Good Birth Project.

The Good Birth Project

At the heart of this book are voices of women who took part in the Good Birth Project, a major study I initiated in 2006 while I was at Duke University. The goal of the project was to develop a full account of what constitutes a good birth, based on a large series of interviews with a diverse group of women who had given birth in a variety of settings, supplemented by interviews with a breadth of maternity care providers.

I designed and carried out the Good Birth Project with concern about birth's dueling mantras and deep curiosity about how women thought about and valued birth. No doubt I'd been around a lot of childbearing women and had attended hundreds of deliveries during residency and my years on the faculty in Duke's general (or "low-risk") obstetrics group. But I hadn't had the opportunity—or perhaps the courage—in short clinic visits to ask the big questions. I knew just a handful of women who'd given birth outside hospitals, and I had a very limited sense of what that experience meant to them. I hadn't attended home births, nor had I ventured into any freestanding birth centers, though one of the country's largest was less than a mile from my house. Over the course of three years, these became familiar conversations and spaces.

I hired a research team and owe a good part of the study's substance and rigor to their careful attention and deftness at interviewing. Taking the lead was anthropologist Emily Namey, who was pregnant for the first time during much of the study. As such, she brought to each interview, along with all the listening and probing skills of an anthropologist, the genuine curiosity of a first-time mom. The result was a mountain of narratives with a profound depth, honesty, and richness of language and meaning.

In choosing whom to interview, it was important to me to cast a broad net—I wanted to hear from a wide range of women with different experiences. So we developed a sampling frame that included women who had given birth in a variety of settings, experienced different modes of delivery, and with a range of maternity care providers. We identified our participants in a variety of ways: flyers posted in local maternity care settings and public places, word of mouth, referrals from midwives and doctors, the Internet. Most were drawn from a metropolitan area served by two large academic medical centers in the southeastern United States, though the births described occurred in geographic regions across the country, in large cities and remote towns. The women we interviewed were diverse in terms of their socioeconomic backgrounds. They gave birth in academic and community hospitals, in birthing centers, and in bathtubs (or not!) at home; eight were transferred from home or a freestanding birthing center to the hospital. Some delivered vaginally with relative ease; some endured emergency cesareans and episiotomies.

About a third of the women were first-time moms, and the rest were seasoned "wise women"—a term we used to refer to women who were looking back on more than one birth. The term has a particular resonance in birth; it has been used to describe certain of those who have traditionally provided help and moral support for women in birth—female relatives, friends, women who had been through birth and have the wisdom of experience to impart. We interviewed first-time moms twice—once toward the end of their pregnancy and once two to six months after delivery; and wise women only once, two to six months after they delivered. We asked everyone to talk about each of their birth experiences, not just the most recent, and encouraged them to speak their minds about whatever they thought relevant. All in all, we heard from 101 women about 196 birth experiences, of which 140 were vaginal, 10 were VBAC (vaginal birth after cesarean), 30 were unplanned cesareans, and 16 were planned cesareans; two cesareans were "elective," meaning there was no accepted medical indication for surgery. Forty-six of the births took place outside a hospital. A detailed table describing the characteristics of the women we interviewed (and their births) can be found in the Appendix.

It was also important to me that we let women talk—that we not impose our views or ways of thinking, that they be allowed to speak in their own words and set their own priorities in their answers. Inspired by psychologist Carol Gilligan's work on moral development (how people evolve with regard to moral reasoning—and differ according to gender), I wanted to hear how women spoke about and valued birth—to get a sense of how they organized their thinking around it, rather than focus on their views about the things we doctors and midwives see as central points of contention. Most of our questions were open-ended. We started by asking women when they thought birth began and when it ended. Then we invited them to tell us, in their own words, about their birth experiences—what made them good, what made them bad, what they'd do differently the next time. Then we probed a short list of topics we were interested in hearing more about. We often asked them to further explain things they said, asking questions like "Why?" and "Can you tell me more about that?" and "What does that word you used mean to you?" We conducted interviews in homes, coffee shops, private rooms in clinics, in a conference room at Duke, on the phone—wherever we could make it work. Newborns were along more often than not, strapped to bodies, sleeping in strollers, getting jiggled, not infrequently punctuating the stories and reflections that poured across their mothers' lips.

In addition to interviewing women about their births, we also interviewed thirty maternity care providers—again they ranged considerably: maternal-fetal specialists; general obstetricians; midwives attending deliveries in hospitals, freestanding birth centers, and homes; labor and delivery nurses and doulas. Several came from the same metropolitan area mentioned above. But our efforts to capture a breadth of views also took us to Washington, D.C.'s Developing Families Center, which houses a freestanding birth center in the heart of the capital's toughest neighborhoods. We also visited the Frontier Nursing University in Kentucky, the oldest and largest continually operating nurse-midwifery school in the United States. And we journeyed to a major nurse-midwifery practice in Lancaster, Pennsylvania. Additional details of how we designed and carried out the study and analyzed the interviews are described in our published work.

What I Found

The birth stories I heard over three years ranged broadly, and were as different as the diverse women we interviewed. But what struck me time and again was not what distinguished one birth from another, but what about them was the same. I was moved by what they had in common despite their differences—even sometimes because of them.

Indeed, there was a striking resonance among the women of the Good Birth Project when they spoke about what mattered in birth—where meaning resided. The themes that emerged cut across home and hospital, and the most straightforward and the most complicated of births. Considered together, what emerged were five primary "domains" related to a good birth experience, including agency, personal security, connectedness, respect, and knowledge, which I discuss in Chapters 2 through 6. One thing that was fascinating is how closely these themes resonate with new accounts of wellbeing, most notably that of ethicists Madison Powers and Ruth Faden in their theory of social justice. But as women's stories suggest, birth demands something particular, something beyond what we hold as good or valuable in life generally. What is needed in birth is not always intuitive or straightforwardly derived from other of life's lessons. In addition, the term and concept of *control* was also mentioned—repeatedly—but didn't seem to have the same explanatory value as the other themes; it seemed to fit into both none and many of the domains. I finally came to see *control* as one of the most important words in birth; I'll explain why in Chapter 1.

One of the hardest parts of translating what I heard to what is in this book was deciding which stories, which women's voices, to portray. Almost every interview was delectably rich, full of nuance, worthy of its own chapter, and full of lessons that would fit nicely in any of them. What I ultimately did was choose *representative* stories—bits of stories sometimes—that portrayed vividly a theme that was echoed by a broad swath of the Good Birth Project's 101 childbearing women and thirty practitioners. They are stories that emblematize shared wisdom. No doubt the births you or your loved ones have experienced (or will experience) will differ in myriad ways from the births you see portrayed here; my hope is that you will find something familiar, authentic, and useful in the wisdom that these particular women have brought to bear. Taken together, their stories paint a nuanced picture of what women really want from childbirth—and they guide us all toward a better understanding of this most profound of experiences.

You will see that these interviews constitute the major threads of the book, but there are other stories, other perspectives represented too. Some are those of colleagues, friends, even strangers (like Elise) moved to share their reflections with me in grocery store aisles and parking lots, on park benches, jogging trails, e-mails, and telephone lines. Others—indeed many—are my own, assembled over the past decade or two as I went from newly minted obstetrician to a more seasoned doctor, from just pregnant in the wake of my father's death to a mother of four and aunt of five more. I have used real names for my family members, but in all other narratives I have changed names and identifying details to maintain confidentiality. The tapestry I've assembled reflects time and experience and offers—I hope—a notion of the good birth that is accessible, familiar, authentic, and empowering; that is both particular and universal; and that is decidedly within reach.

Why a Good Birth Matters

When I first started this book, I was often met with excitement (and birth stories). But every once in a while I was met with skepticism, or even hostility. "Tell me, Annie, why does it matter?" the skeptical friend or colleague, or even a stranger, would ask. "Why do we make such a big deal of the 'birth experience'—shouldn't a healthy baby be enough?"

My initial response was to bristle, take offense—not just for myself but for women, my patients, my friends. But those who ask the question why have women in mind as well. The worry is that this "good birth" is potentially just another thing for women to beat themselves up about. No doubt idealizing a certain sort of birth has left too many women feeling disappointed, feeling like they didn't live up to an ideal. And that is a pretty rotten way to begin one of the biggest jobs of your life.

I appreciate that the alternative to my approach would be to jettison the idea of a good birth altogether and quit focusing on experience. To reorient toward birth's ends, perhaps leaving us to focus on how to prioritize health outcomes.

So if at first blush confused and offended by those who ask, "Why does it matter?" I have come to take it to be a fair question. And I have four answers, or reasons, why the pursuit of a good birth matters.

The first reason is that women matter. Since you are reading this book, perhaps I don't need to make this argument. But perhaps I do. Birth is not just about babies; it is not just an occasion in which a child enters the world. It is an occasion in which women turn into mothers (and men into fathers; more on this below). It is a time in which our hearts stretch, our priorities shift, our view of the world is transformed. *We* are transformed. This is a point I'll discuss in the book's final chapter, but I think it worth noting at the outset.

There is a view that we mothers should be grateful and, perhaps more to the point, satisfied with the simple fact that we have brought healthy children into the world (or some would argue, any children into the world, whatever their health status). But there is a problem with that view—it erases us, our experience, *our* transformation. As mother of two Molly put it, "Just to say that a healthy baby is the only important thing kind of reduces women down to being baby machines. Like, what, they don't matter? I don't like that at all."

I don't like it either. But I've made a research career out of countering what my dear friend and colleague Ruth Faden has termed the "vessels and vectors" problem: the tendency of even the well intentioned to focus on fetuses and children in research studies, ethical analyses, and conversations, and forget about the women in whose bodies they are growing and whose lives they will shape. In 1985, esteemed professor of public health Allan Rosenfield highlighted that so-called maternal and child health or MCH programs had focused primarily on children's health, their presumption being that what's good for a baby is good for a mother. But the programs gave almost no attention to maternal health as an end itself, leading Rosenfield and his coauthor to ask, "Where is the M in MCH?" A decade later, Faden called attention to the fact that the vast efforts to conduct research on HIV considered women only in their capacity to infect their children or their intimate partners. Another decade passed, and the same problem remained. In 2008, the National Institutes of Health rolled out a major study involving 100,000 pregnant women in order to examine how the environment affects health; data were collected almost exclusively as they related to these women's children. The women—the participants in research—were part of the "environment" to be studied rather than people about whom we might learn something.

Certainly there are forces—social, cultural, psychological perhaps— that make women's importance feel—even to women at times—like a matter of contention; that turn the attention of even well-intentioned doctors and midwives, policy makers, and researchers away from childbearing women as subjects themselves. But giving birth is a major life event; if birth marks the entry of a new person into the world, the fact of and interests of the person who made it happen are well worth our attention.

My mother has always been pretty fabulous about making her children and grandchildren feel celebrated on their birthdays. Even when I was in college and residency, she'd make sure the day felt special and I felt adored. If I was on call, she made sure to get in touch—it was one of the few times she'd navigate the complex call system, greet the operator, and ask to talk to me. And I knew when I got home the next morning there would be something on the doorstep. A gorgeous bouquet with my favorite snapdragons, or an artfully wrapped package enclosing something she knew I'd love. But since my children's births, I've started to think that the attention should flow in the other direction. That I should make sure I call my mother on my birthday (not just on hers)—and perhaps that I beat her to it. For a birthday, it strikes me, is an occasion to celebrate not just the child but the mother, the person for whom that day was in other ways the start of things, a beginning, a birth.

Of course there are others who are so changed by birth—fathers, for starters. For many men, birth is an experience, hopefully good and undoubtedly transformative. Birth can be exhilarating, scary, alienating, deeply memorable for anyone intimately involved. No doubt my own dad's response to his children's births is one reason I've been so riveted by the process. Still, it is women who give birth, whose bodies are breached by it, and who, it always strikes me, are or should be the primary subjects of childbirth, even as it marks the lives of those around them and shifts their relationships. The experiences of partners and other loved ones deserve attention, to be sure, and other researchers and scholars have made important progress in this regard. But in shaping a new conception of the good birth, I draw primarily upon the wisdom of childbearing women and speak in particular to their childbirth experience.

This brings me to the second reason that we should care about and pursue the good birth: birth matters to women.

For one, memories of birth have a certain tenacity—they endure, they stay with us. Women remember their births, often vividly, whether good or bad. Author Joyce Maynard once famously wrote, "I think of my children's births—carry them around with me—every day of my life." Not everyone feels this way, but some people do. Doula, childbirth educator, and author Penny Simkin actually studied women's memories of birth, and found that years after a birth (meaning double digits), women's memories are "generally accurate and strikingly vivid." Notably, Simkin found that the physical and clinical features of labor emerged as less important than the way women remembered being treated and how they remembered acting and feeling. She reports these findings in a series of two articles, aptly titled, "Just Another Day in a Woman's Life?"

Simkin's findings are hardly surprising. All the women we interviewed for the Good Birth Project had had a baby within six months of the interview, but those who had given birth more than once could recall with striking clarity births that happened years before. When I've mentioned the project in conversations with friends and strangers, recollections are similarly vivid, and as you will see became a rich source of information for my book. Whatever their age or distance in time from giving birth, women (and sometimes men) will disclose details of the event—how their child looked at them, what was said, how it felt.

Further, birth is a source not just of memories but of *meaning*; it is a big piece of how birth matters to women. Birth can be a way to claim (or reclaim) a sense of power. It can be a self-test, a form of resistance to things that impose on, constrain, or threaten us, and it can be a way to heal from loss.

No doubt this meaning bit can get out of hand. For one, it presses some women toward choices that I'd call ill-advised; it can distract in ways that are dangerous or destructive, and can be fertile ground for judgment. I worried about it last year, when two of my good friends from college had babies—very differently—at the time. One gave birth at home and was immensely proud, while the other had a complicated hospital birth and looked back at it with feelings of regret. I worried when they took a trip together what it would mean for their friendship, whether there might be a sliding from pride to judgment, from disappointment to shame or resentment. In the end, the friendship endured. They shared their stories, their children. The way they gave birth didn't define them, but it sure made them wiser, and they were good enough friends to tell each other how. For those who need an interlocutor and a framework upon which to hang their wisdom or to regard that of others, *A Good Birth*—I trust—will fit the bill.

Third, birth matters because it's the beginning of a story, of a life and the relationships that shape it, and beginnings matter to us—all of us.

Until my boys were about six or so, there was a game we played when I pulled them out of the tub. We had those hooded towels that imparted visages of creatures, and once I'd wrapped up each boy, they'd curl up on the bath mat underneath the terry-cloth spikes of a stegosaurus or fin of a shark.

"Sit on me!" they'd clamor, and holding on to the edge of the tub I'd sit on their backs, and the game would begin. I was the mommy dinosaur, sitting on an egg, imagining out loud just how wonderful my babies would be when they hatched. Then rumble-crack-crack—the terry-cloth mound would start to move and giggle—and lo and behold, out would emerge the naked boy, the baby dinosaur, and I'd tell him how delighted and overjoyed I was that he had arrived, how wonderful it was to finally meet him.

I've started to wonder at the reptilian game—why we started it, why it caught on. My boys, after all, know the difference between mammals and their egg-laying relatives. One of my friends told me she did more mammalian-themed creation stories with her girls, enlisting the quilt on the bed as the costume of pregnancy, their emergence from beneath it as their birth. The exchange once they'd arrived was very much the same. We all care about how birth goes; it's the beginning of a life together, chapter one of a story that is—one hopes—a love affair to boot.

Indeed, author Louise Erdrich has called labor itself "both a paradigm and parable."

> The story of the body becomes a touchstone, a predictor. A mother or father, in describing their labor, relates the personality of the child to some piece of the event, makes the story into a frame, an introduction, a prelude to the child's life, molds the labor into the story that is no longer a woman's story or a man's story, but the story of a child.

Birth is a serious, momentous event—serious and momentous not just for the person who is born but for the person who gives birth. It is an event of human importance, an event that holds for many of us bodily and existential meaning. Perhaps that alone marks why getting it right—getting to the good—is a critical project.

Fourth, the health care landscape is changing rapidly and with it birth practices. There are 4.3 million births per year in the United States, and their impact on the health care system is significant: 23 percent of all women discharged from hospitals have just given birth; six of the fifteen most common hospital procedures involve childbirth; and more than a quarter of all procedures performed on women are obstetrical. Maternal and newborn hospital charges were $86 billion in 2006, far exceeding those of any other condition. It is not surprising, then, that maternity care has garnered scrutiny and is likely to continue to do so in the context of health care reform.

Yet given the polarized dialogue between midwifery and obstetrics, efforts to improve maternity care have been stymied by divergent views about the nature of quality and the goals of care. This is likely to continue in the absence of a grounded understanding of how childbearing women view quality in the context of birth. Women's voices should inform measures to evaluate and improve the quality of care. Without a grounded understanding of what makes for a good birth experience, it will be difficult to develop measures of how well we are doing, and to determine whether maternity care is moving in the right direction.

Furthermore, our continued divisions over approaches to birth can put women in harm's way. Professionals' views of birth have resulted in insufficient collaboration in the care of birthing women, although practitioners and women alike stand to benefit from the synergies professional partnerships would entail. When doctors and midwives argue, it is often women who lose: women transferred from home to hospital, women who value both the intimacies championed by midwifery and ready access to modern technologies. Women's voices highlight areas of shared value for professionals, shifting the dialogue away from technology and pathology, and toward considerations that matter most to women. My hope is that this dialogue will draw on the strengths of *both* medically oriented obstetrics and midwifery, and lead to professional partnerships that will facilitate efficient, high-quality, patient-centered maternity care.

We're not going to unseat the quest for a good birth. Birth has been a source of scrutiny, debate, and meaning-making across cultures and through-out history. And so my approach has been try to recraft an understanding of the good that doesn't leave women feeling ashamed, that doesn't add fuel to the fires of judgment, that gives women a framework for understanding what matters to them in birth, so they can have the experiences they want, and value the experiences they get.

How to Use This Book

This book proposes a new frame through which to view birth. It is organized around the things women say they found to be most important in birth.

I try not to take sides: I won't argue for any particular place for or ap-proach to birth. Rather, my goals with this book are to offer a new way of thinking about this important life event and to provide guideposts for navi-gating the choices you may face approaching birth and the challenges to un-derstanding and valuing birth that may occur in its wake.

Sometimes I'll offer practical steps you can take in service of the things women say are valuable—things that can be done, for instance, to maintain what feels like respectful or sacred space in birth. Other times I'll offer a back story—let you in as best I can to what goes on in the hearts and minds of people (like doctors) who care for women in birth. And most of the time, I'll pull apart something that is generally tussled or fretted about and help you understand what's at the heart of the matter, paving the way for you to under-stand what it might mean in your situation. My hope is that this book leaves you feeling not just wiser but more empowered as you plan your birth experience.

I wrote this book, for the most part, with mothers and mothers-to-be in mind. So you will see that much of the advice I distill is directed toward them (or you, as the case may be). And when I say mothers, I refer not just to those looking toward their next birth, but also to the many mothers for whom birthing will never happen again but whom I hope to help find ways to better understand and find the goodness in the births they have had. And I also refer to grandmothers and grandmothers-to-be—the "wise women" who can be wiser still in supporting younger women whom they love in their birthing experiences. But there are also lessons in here for fathers and partners, doctors and midwives, advocates and policy makers, observers and shapers of birth in the myriad ways people can be. Many such lessons are assembled in the epilogue, though you will also find them throughout the text—sometimes marked explicitly as directives to partners, loved ones, providers; other lessons depend on our curiosity, our empathy, our willingness to imagine what we would do, or want, if we were giving birth.

I offer two final caveats before we begin.

First, there is an understandable tendency to link birth and motherhood—to imagine that birth and how "well" you do it determine what sort of mom you will be, that it is the first of many tests—and a nerve-racking one at that. But what I hope you'll take from this book is something very different. Birth is an end in itself. It is not a test, not a measure of worth. But it is and will always be an important moment in women's lives, and this book and the women whose voices populate its pages are an effort to tell us how—to tell us why, really, a good birth matters.

It's important too—because any discussion of a "good" birth can threaten to make it sound like the terms of a test. But my point in identifying shared themes, things that women say are deeply at issue in birth, is not to give a template of "the" good birth any more than prior efforts to identify the same sorts of themes around what matters at the end of life have had as their end a template for "the" good death. All births, like all deaths, are different—and finding the good in either is particular to the person going through it.

Second, any number of births that are lacking in one or more of the elemental qualities women identify as so important can be deeply meaningful—even profound, for all that. Herein lies the most profound lesson of the Good Birth Project, and of my book. As I hinted above, the link between birth and death will be a theme throughout, and it does its best work in answering this challenge. If life's final passage has the potential to be as full of beauty and meaning as life's first, I think the analogy also works in the opposite direction—that birth is also like death, in many ways, but pointedly because both inevitably involve loss. But it is not a bad kind of loss, necessarily. We lose our former self, and in its place we become mothers; we lose the ideal baby we'd imagined, and in its place we get the baby we will love; we lose an idealized birth experience, and in its place we get something real, something full of beauty, something that is our very own.

I've been told that whenever the Amish make a quilt, they leave an imperfection, a flaw. Historians argue over its meaning and some even question its intentionality, but the quilt served as a powerful analogy for me as I thought through the lessons of the Good Birth Project. Just like the quilts, our births won't be perfect, or meet an idealized notion of the good (neither will we, nor will our children), but therein lies our humanity, and that, I would argue, is where we find beauty and meaning. The imperfection (the disrespectful word, the moment of terror, the tussle with control) doesn't mean that all will unravel (not the quilt, our births, ourselves), but rather that we are firmly in the world. The goal is not the ideal birth, not the perfect birth, but the Good Birth, after all.

one

Control

*Perhaps my greatest stroke of luck was penetrating quickly to the central
paradox of childbirth: that the only way to gain control is to lose it, and that
the courage to name the pain must precede the courage to bear it.*

—SUSAN MAUSHART

*There are certain frustrations in approaching such an event, a drama in
which the body stars and not the fiction-making mind. In a certain way, I'm
jealous. I want to control the tale. I can't—therein lies the conflict that
drives this plot in the first place.*

—LOUISE ERDRICH

There is (or will be) a time in pregnancy when you'll feel it—that flutter, that
bubble, that sensation that you know is something other than yourself.
Something, someone, under your skin—a part of you, but not quite—over
which you have little control but immense responsibility.

It's something I've become accustomed to over the years, over pregnancies, losses, and births—my own and those of others for whom I've cared.
But it never ceases to move me. When I was writing the first draft of this
chapter, pregnant with now one-year-old William, there it was: as I gazed
over my pregnant belly to type, a sudden protrusion—perhaps a heel or an
elbow—reminding me that I was not fully "in control" of my pregnancy, of
my body, of William's impending birth.

Maybe you will remember it in its first iteration—that initial moment of
"quickening" (as the first sensations of fetal movement were once called).
For me it was vivid, feeling a baby under the skin for the first time. I can still

picture the tile pattern in the bathroom where I sat, the shortness and deepness of the tub, the water made tepid in the spirit of gestational caution. Seared in mind like a handful of other moments, like moments in which you hear news—good or bad—that will change your life, the world, or both.

Or maybe it will come upon you as a slow rumble, a gradual realization as the protrusions across your belly become more pronounced. Or suddenly at the end of your pregnancy, when you give birth; or when your child is in your arms, in your new line of sight. It's not just the fact of the baby I'm talking about. It is, rather, the way that pregnancy and birth bring control—both its importance and elusiveness—into sharp relief.

Control has turned out to be one of the most common—and vexing—terms I've encountered over my years of discussing childbirth, whether chatting with another mom, asking a patient what she wants from her birth experience, or interviewing women for the Good Birth Project. Indeed, almost half the women my team and I interviewed spontaneously mentioned the word *control* in their discussions, and many more affirmed its importance when we asked them about it. They said that they felt out of control during birth; that they wanted more control; that they appreciated that a certain obstetrician or midwife let them take control; that holding on, in some way, to control as they understood it was "very important" to a good birth. Others have noticed this too: in a comprehensive review of studies measuring "satisfaction" in birth, nurse and researcher Ellen Hodnett found control and childbirth satisfaction to be strongly related. And as you'll see in this chapter and throughout the book, so much of a good birth ties back to the notion of control.

But women of the Good Birth Project also say, "Not so fast." They tell us that a good birth requires letting go of control, sometimes because you have to, but sometimes because it feels like you should. They spoke of the strangeness of choosing a delivery date, of knowing their baby's sex, of taking charge of (or responsibility for) a physiologically uncontrollable process. "You can't control birth," we heard time and again—and from some, there was a resistance to the idea that you should even try.

In trying to reconcile these two views, I've come to regard *control* as one of the most important words in birth, a key to understanding what we're after. But finding control requires knowing what it means, the ways in which it's important, and how it's related to the good in birth, for you.

Letting Go

Let's begin with those mixed feelings about control. Again, while women often brought it up themselves and talked about how important control was, they further told us that letting go—ceding control—was also key to a good birth.

The importance of letting go was something that many women discovered over time. It was a lesson, hard wrought for some. "Don't try and control it, because you can't," mother of two Melissa advised. In her first birth, labor caught her by surprise two weeks early, and she was "just kind of open to whatever happened." The next time around, she went past her due date and got to plan everything, down to the doctor, the day, the approach to initiating labor.

"I'm a control freak," she told us, "so it actually surprises me that I enjoyed my first birth more, where I wasn't trying to control everything, where I was going with the flow." The second time around, when she was ostensibly "in control," she said she felt like she missed out on something, on "some kind of the magic of the birth experience."

My friend Geri came to a similar conclusion as she reflected on her first birth, the story of which spilled out over a cup of coffee we recently shared. Geri is a powerful executive, widely admired for her command of her field, her company, the delicate balance struck between work and life—for the way she has always seemed to be "in control." But, she told me, her first birth shifted indelibly her relationship to control and the ways in which it could be hers—in all of life no less than in childbirth.

At the time of her first birth, she was a thirty-year-old lawyer who, only two weeks before her due date, had just argued the most contentious hearing of her career. The judge had ruled against her—and adding insult to injury, had asked her to draft his proposed order in the matter. "Usually that job went to the victors," she told me, "but it was the 1980s, and chauvinism still reigned, so I got stuck with it." Hot, irritated—and unbeknownst to her, contracting—but determined to press on, she drove back to her office to tackle the pile of work that awaited her.

She stayed at work through the day and decided to take the subway home, even though she was feeling worse. She wasn't about to give in to the draw of an expensive cab, and instead carefully choreographed an onboard meeting with her husband, who got on at a different subway stop. (This was a feat that only master schedulers like Geri could accomplish in the era before cell phones.)

Then came the first hint that control as she knew it was going to change, and her birth was going to be the catalyst: as she triumphantly stepped through the subway door and waved hello to her husband, she remembered she had driven to work that day. "What was happening to me?" she recalled thinking. "Where was my brain? We took the subway back to my office to get my car, drove home, and when I stood up to get out of the car, it happened. My mucus plug—a wet seat. 'Oh my God,' I thought. I was delivering two weeks early."

Her first impulse was to hold on, to keep on the tracks of the day she'd planned. "I had to lecture to three hundred people the next day about preparing a will. How was I going to do that? I looked at my watch. Still early evening. A quick labor, an easy delivery, I would be out by . . . no, was I crazy? Someone else would have to do the lecture. But there was still time to do the order! Between contractions, I furiously scribbled it all onto a pad of paper and dictated it to my colleague over the phone. I ended our conversation by begging him to do the lecture, then hung up."

The ride to the doctor's office and then the hospital was excruciating, as her plans for drug-free birth flew out the window. "When I got to the hospital," she said, "I wanted drugs and wanted them *now*." But the epidural she requested did next to nothing for her pain, and only seemed to slow down her labor. It felt to her like the perfect capstone to a day of what she called "failed plans."

Five hours later, however, Geri had given birth, her daughter Brett was in her arms, and suddenly none of the day's twists and turns seemed to matter. "As I looked down at her," she said, "it hit me: I had just said good-bye to control, and it was never coming back. I was now out of control for the rest of my life. But I didn't care. I couldn't have been happier."

That day, Geri realized something that many women of the Good Birth Project echoed in their interviews: "You can't control birth." Strictly speaking, they are right. No matter what scientific inroads we make, we cannot predict with certainty the hour or the day our babies will arrive—even those who plan a "scheduled cesarean" may be surprised. Nor can we assure ourselves that gestation and delivery will go smoothly or according to plan. We can't orchestrate the actions of our loved ones or caregivers; the ones we handpick might not even make it there—whether our ob-gyn is off call or the midwife's car breaks down on the way to the birth center. We (thankfully) won't be able to control what our children look like or who they are. Childbirth can make a mockery of the best-laid plans.

No doubt this can be a source of frustration for women who expect the alternative. Control is part of the mantra of modern reproduction: women's liberation is based in large part on our ability to control when we get pregnant, or at least when we do not. The idea of control has permeated other parts of our lives as well. From navigating traffic patterns to hearing a favorite song with a few swipes on a palm-size device, we have the means to fine-tune our days. So it's no surprise that many women heading toward birth think about control as a good thing, something to which we should unabashedly aspire. And many presume that—if we go to the right birthing classes, pick the right practitioner, download the right app (complete with weight tracker, kick counter, and contraction timer), understand well enough how to breathe—we can indeed "control" our birth and that, as with other things in our life, with enough preparation it will unfold as envisioned. But the fact of the matter is that it rarely does.

The other day I bumped into Kelly, a good friend of mine from residency, now an incredibly popular obstetrician in town. I was a couple of years ahead of her in training, so I often supervised her in the ever-hierarchical system, and it was always a pleasure. When we worked together, she was top in her game—and still is when it comes to practicing obstetrics. Not just smart and capable, but utterly organized—calmly, pleasantly obsessive. Coming to work any morning that Kelly had been overseeing Labor and Delivery the night before meant we'd be drinking coffee by ten (rather than grabbing a doughnut at four), since she'd have everything—and everyone—in such perfect order for the morning obstetrics team. She got things done, but was sweet about it; patients loved her. On top of all that, she was trim and gorgeous, by virtue of the fact that she always found time to work in a run—before a long shift or after. If anyone exuded control during the oppressiveness that was residency training, it was Kelly.

But Kelly faced her own challenges after residency was over. She was diagnosed with breast cancer in her early thirties—and again her style was decisive, in control. She wasn't going to let cancer take over. Based on what she knew of herself and the disease, she chose to undergo a bilateral mastectomy and get a "new rack" instead of enduring radiation as her oncologist recommended. When ten years later the cancer was decidedly at bay, she got pregnant with twins.

I recently saw her at the pool with her boys—now just over two. She was her composed, "in control" self, as evidenced by the fact we could actually talk while she was watching and gently managing two wild little towheads, who couldn't swim, at the edge of the pool. But, she told me, giving birth to them was a lesson in control and its limits.

Kelly labored at thirty-one weeks, nine weeks early. When she got to the hospital, she told me, "I was out of control." She screamed at the young doctor who checked her in and told her she was fully dilated ("You are wrong!"), at the anesthesiologist who placed her epidural ("Knock me out!"), and yes, at her husband, whom she adored. And you must understand—I'd seen Kelly pressed to the wall before. She was invariably calm when a patient's life was in the balance, when absorbing the verbal impalement that none of us completely escaped during residency training, when she was told she'd have to stay on call another twenty-four hours because her replacement was sick. No doubt residency was hard. But this—birth—was different.

"I feel like birth was my comeuppance," she ultimately reflected. "Now I get it, all those screaming women I've seen in the middle of the night, over the years. I was one of them now." Birth, Kelly concluded, was not a marathon or residency or anything like either. Birth could not be planned or controlled. It would not be micromanaged.

But is micromanagement what we really want? According to the women of the Good Birth Project, no. Like Geri and Kelly, most women come to understand that they do cede a certain amount of control when they go into labor—not just to caregivers, but to their bodies, nature, even fate perhaps. It doesn't determine whether they think their birth was good or not. Rather, it becomes something that shifts the way they understand what's possible, what birth—and the good birth—entails.

Banker Stephanie, thirty-seven, spoke of weeping in the delivery room at an uncanny realization before her birth that control, as she knew it, was gone, that birth brought with it the demand for a certain sort of "surrender."

> To finally be at this moment when you've waited so long . . . I mean, it was kind of stunning. I remember sitting in the delivery room and looking at the place where they put the baby and thinking, "This is it." I was crying, and my husband was like, "Well, you wanted a baby," and I said, "I know I want the baby," but I was just very emotional.
>
> I think that there's probably little control [laughs] in birth, and I think that that's why I started to cry with [my first], because it was just going to happen. It was like, "There's no going back. . . . But it is, for a type-A person, for a firstborn, it is very unnerving. It's probably one of the only times in my life that I felt like this is happening and there is not much I can do about it. It's almost like a surrender.

Yet for Stephanie—who went on to speak without regret of a wonderful birth—and many others, control's elusiveness did not ruin the experience. Stephanie is one of the mothers who tell us that a good birth embraces the uncanny; a good birth is not about scheduling, about picking a birthday or doctor or even a method of delivery.

In fact, many women found something strange, even ill-conceived in having control over certain things, like dictating the time and place of delivery. Such was the case with twenty-nine-year-old Emma, who spoke about how odd it felt to schedule birth, as she did when she learned her baby would need to be delivered via cesarean.

> The weird part [was] determining [my] baby's birthday; I think
> that's very odd. We knew it was going to be in the second week
> of March. My doctor was like, "How does it work into your
> schedule? This day or this day?" . . . Back in September we knew
> that he was going to be born on the sixteenth of March.

Scheduling delivery can feel arbitrary or trivial; it can feel like negotiating with the universe for something beyond our power to determine. Undergirding our discomfort is the idea that you shouldn't control birth—that doing so would be tempting fate. That having too much control of when or even how birth happens is, as mother of two Lisa put it, "playing with fire." Picking a delivery date, she reflected, is "a little more control than anybody should have."

Part of Emma's and Lisa's reluctance to control isn't completely rational, as they themselves acknowledge. The baby will come whether we pick the day or not, and the act of choosing is unlikely to affect the outcome. The worry is about the hands of fate—that if we exert too much control, we are messing with the cosmos, with the predictions or the stars. Still, the paradox surrounding control is fascinatingly clear here: we want control, and yet we don't—at least not too much, or the wrong kind of control.

In listening to women's stories, there was also what struck me as an entirely rational argument for not controlling birth. It's not just about averting frustration (which I'd also count as rational). It's that ambivalence (or rejection) of control was in service of the good birth, that letting go can be *what makes it good*. Many women will talk about how powerful it felt to have their body "take over"—to recognize that birth was happening, and there was nothing they, or anyone, could do about it. Many, like Abby, found it awe-inspiring. She delivered her daughter in the backseat of her car, and described with excitement the feeling that she wasn't in control, that her baby was coming and there wasn't a thing she could do about it. "It wasn't like I could cross my legs," she remembered. "It was like there was something deep down, something primitive telling me what to do." She ripped off her pants and pulled her daughter out of her body and onto her chest (while her husband, gaping, watched through the car's window). It wasn't what she had envisioned, but each time she recounts the story, her blue eyes sparkle.

In the end, ceding control isn't giving up. Women who celebrate giving birth, who are empowered before or because of childbirth, cede control; and they'll tell you that it's constructive, necessary, part and parcel of the good birth. Part of getting ready for birth is understanding this: it's not just planning for the sort of birth you hope for, but getting used to the idea, the necessity, of letting go.

Holding On

A good birth is not *just* about ceding control, however. Instead, as seasoned nurse-midwife Donna told us, there is a "happy medium" when it comes to control. "If a woman comes in and wants to be in total control," she told us, "she's not going to have it. But if a woman abdicates and gives all her control to someone else, she's not going to have it either." By "it," I think Donna was talking about the sort of control that *is* important to a good birth, something to which you should hold fast—that elusive notion that trips up so many of us the first time (or first couple of times) around. Control continues to hold a valuable place in a good birth.

For mothers a good birth is one that gives us a sense that we can contain the uncertainty that childbearing entails—that we can in some way *preside* over birth and maintain a sense of integrity as we ride its uncontrollable wake. As midwife Amy put it, "It's not really controlling the process as much as it is hanging on as you are going through it, this roller-coaster ride of labor and birth." But how?

The Expectations Fallacy

Some people assume that the key is expectations—that a good birth depends on having expectations met. They think that the sort of control that makes a birth good can be found in a combination of informed planning and (realistically) some luck, of knowing what you can control and planning *that*. Indeed, millions of women have been led to believe that what is key is knowing "what to expect."

In some ways, it makes sense. To be pregnant is of course to be *expecting*—literally, to anticipate, to look forward. Pregnant women are *expectant* mothers. Any woman anticipating birth will think about what her birth will be like. During the course of pregnancy, she will undoubtedly receive solicited and unsolicited accounts of birth experiences from friends and acquaintances (and sometimes strangers), may see depictions of or actual births on television, and may seek out reading materials or a childbirth education class to answer questions and become "prepared." Whether actively sought or not, the stories and advice begin shaping our expectations about everything from pain, to pain management, to desired birth location and delivery mode. And for women having a second or subsequent baby, their previous experience(s) contribute to more concrete desires and expectations about how their upcoming birth will go.

In light of the emphasis on expectations, it's not surprising that many of the doctors and midwives we talked to pinpointed expectations as the key to a good birth. Some focused on women's expectations for *outcome*: "If your only expectation is that 'My baby is healthy,' then most women are very pleased, because regardless of what we do, they get a healthy baby," offered Scott, an obstetrician we interviewed. The more careful and responsive among them also brought up women's expectations about *process*. But in their understandable focus on expectations, these providers miss the point. If women who get what they wanted are often satisfied, the births that veer from said expectations (and they are the majority) are not necessarily less good because they entailed the unexpected. Thus the "control" that wise women say is important to a good birth can't simply be understood as having a birth go according to plan.

Two women's stories help me illustrate this last point. At first glance, their births were strikingly similar. Both had planned a hospital birth with epidural anesthesia. Both entered birth invested in and trusting of the medical establishment: Wren was herself a nurse, Liz was married to a fellow in cardiology, and both were unabashedly counting on the field to deliver anesthesia safely and swiftly.

As it turned out, neither Wren nor Liz got the epidural they wanted, though each requested one (repeatedly) on arrival at the hospital. Both were laboring hard when they reached the Labor and Delivery ward; both were assured that an anesthesiologist had been alerted; each had to wait several

hours to see one, and both ultimately delivered their babies before an epidural could be placed.

What distinguished the two women—and profoundly—was their assessment of the birth after the fact. For Wren—who before the experience
had said, "I'm a nurse. I know the beauty of drugs, okay? . . . There's no gold
medals for having natural childbirth"—the unexpected turn of events was
"extremely positive . . . fabulous," and she felt "extremely empowered." Liz,
though, assessed her birth overall as "very negative" and was "extremely
disappointed in the whole hospital."

Clearly, it's not about expectations being met—neither woman's were. I
can vouch that it wasn't about personality, either; both Wren and Liz are
clear-eyed, pragmatic people not given to ready enthusiasm or complaining.
So what was different? What made Wren's birth fabulous and Liz's terrible?
Let's take a closer look.

For one, Wren's story is replete with connections forged over the course
of her labor. She describes the nurse who met her on the Labor and Delivery
ward, who acknowledged her and the intensity of her experience.

> My nurse's name—I'll never forget her name. She's a real tall
> black lady with big hair piled on top of her head. She had tons of
> jewelry on. And she hooked me up to the monitor and she
> kept saying, once she looked at my contractions, she was like,
> "Whoa, fast and furious. Your contractions are coming fast and
> furious."

When it came time to push, Wren described her exchange with another
nurse, who helped bring her from a place of fear to empowerment.

> I had pure fear. I had never for once in my whole pregnancy
> thought I would go through it without drugs . . . And I remem-
> ber looking over at her—I said, "What do I do?" And she just
> gave me a smile and she said, "You grab both your knees and
> push." I said, "Okay, I'll do that." And she, like, was very
> matter-of-fact, which is what I needed.

Liz's story, on the other hand, was marked by a pervasive theme of abandonment and isolation. Over the course of her hospital stay, her trust in and connectedness to her providers began to fall apart.

> [I was] laboring in this little triage room. Nobody—no epidural, no anesthesiologist—really, I saw the doctor twice and the nurse maybe two or three times. Waiting. Okay. And this keeps continuing . . . from seven to now it's ten-thirty. I finally get into a Labor and Delivery room. I almost felt like I was sort of lied to, because I kept asking and they kept saying I was going to get into a labor room, and they kept saying I was going to get an epidural, and all these hours had passed and none of that had happened.

When Liz arrived in the labor room, she (like Wren) was also afraid, most centrally at a moment when the nurse could not find her baby's heart rate. But in sharp contrast to what we heard from Wren stands Liz's description of the moment—of a profound sense of isolation.

> I'm feeling very much out of control. And at that point my doctor wasn't there. There was an anesthesiologist, there was a resident I had never met, there was a nurse who was wonderful, and some other people I didn't know. My husband was off in the corner, couldn't see him . . . and I was just looking around at all of these people I didn't know and knowing that they couldn't find my baby's heartbeat.

For Liz, the unmet expectation—not receiving an epidural for the bulk of her labor—was certainly one reason for her disappointment with her birth, but what truly made the birth a bad experience was being left alone, uninformed or "lied to," and feeling disconnected from the providers who did attend her, resulting in her perception that things were "out of control"—that she was out of control. She does, like Wren, mention the presence of one "wonderful" nurse, but in this case, even an attentive and supportive nurse could not make up for what was lacking.

What Wren's and Liz's stories make clear is that there is more to a good birth than having things go according to plan. Wren and Liz didn't simply want the births they expected; they wanted the emotional satisfaction, security, and connectedness that they imagined would have been available by virtue of the plans they made. But there are many ways to achieve these things whether or not all the boxes on their expectations checklist had been ticked. The sort of control that women value in birth is not simply about getting what they planned or expected. And that, ultimately, is why I chose to start *A Good Birth* by talking about control. If its meaning is hard to pin down, it is nevertheless an umbrella under which so much that we care about in birth resides.

As we begin to peer under that umbrella, it's worth taking an even deeper look at control itself. Why does it mean so much to us in the first place? In what ways are our desires for control competing with our doctors' or midwives' desires for control, and why? Obviously, if you are approaching birth, you aren't going to change your doctor or midwife (though you'd be surprised about how moved we can be). I'm telling you these things so you can get a better sense of the landscape, the forces that I think move us in the delivery room to act in ways that may be confusing or alarming, and in books and other public spaces to argue or advocate for certain ways—*our* ways—of doing things. It's a way for you to get a better sense of what's beneath the birth wars and the behaviors of the people who provide care in birth for you or someone you care about. Ultimately, by exploring these questions, you can get a sense of the ways in which a good birth does depend on control, and how it is that you can meaningfully and productively hold on.

Doctors, Midwives, and the Whys of Control

It wasn't long ago when women didn't have a choice in the delivery room, when control wasn't an option. Midwife Kitty Ernst has called mid-century obstetrics the "knock 'em out, drag 'em out days" when heavy sedation and forceps were the norm. Kitty blasted off as an advocate for women after she saw that version of obstetrics firsthand as a student nurse in the

1940s—births in which she told us women were "out of control" by virtue of the fact that they were given the drug scopolamine and often tied to the bed so—as she tells it—they wouldn't hurt themselves. These were days in which control was utterly elusive, when women didn't get to decide about much of anything when they entered the hospital in labor.

If birth practices have improved, many doctors still feel a need for control in labor rooms. "We are physicians," Alison, a general obstetrician reflected, "because we like to be in control. And I think a lot of times [when we're] taking care of people who also want control, we can lock horns and get into power struggles."

Some have blamed doctors' urge to control birth on disrespect—even hatred—of women. If a doctor's manner stems in any way, shape, or form from latent misogyny, from his need to assert power or his lack of respect for women's rights to dominion over their bodies or reproductive lives, his actions deserve nothing but condemnation. But to understand birth debates merely in terms of empowered women versus overbearing doctors is to miss a good part of what's going on.

For control in birth will come up even for staunch advocates of women. In residency, colleagues and I used to bristle at the "swagger"—you see it among some scrub-clad obstetricians who hold themselves with a certain air when they have forceps in hand. Forceps are the instruments appropriately used to effect delivery when the pushing stage has been too long or its continuation is a threat to the health of a woman or her infant. But if it is frightening and unsettling to imagine large metal tongs placed around the sweet head of one's child, forceps have what you might call a bad rap with feminists and maternity care advocates for other reasons entirely. In tracing the history of forceps in her classic *Of Woman Born*, Adrienne Rich called them the "masculine weapon" in the public struggle between male surgeons and female midwives in the 1700s (interestingly, she also wondered whether midwives of the time would have condemned them so sweepingly if their use had been permitted to women). Contemporary advocates have continued the critique, casting forceps as instruments of male power—of communicating, as anthropologist Robbie Davis-Floyd puts it, "superiority and control of Male over Female, Technology over Nature."

Perhaps that is still how forceps are experienced by some swaggering doctors and their (unfortunate) patients. No doubt they are harmful in the hands of a few. But a good many doctors of both sexes have a different sense of them. Having learned from the most gentle and competent in my field how to use them, access to forceps is as reassuring to me as any of obstetrics' tools. They can impart a sense that one has in hand what it takes to get a baby into the world; to pull when pushes won't suffice; to get through the hand-wringing and feelings of powerlessness that can accompany a protracted labor. I've used them to ease out a distressed baby when the only other option for delivery would have been an emergency cesarean; I've used them to help a tired mom deliver vaginally, triumphantly. Forceps and other technologies are not necessarily weapons against women but a bulwark of sorts against the caprices of birth. My sense is that some patients see them that way too. My dear college friend Sydney exuded only relief at her doctor's application and confident use of the instruments in the delivery of her first (and large-headed) child after she'd been pushing for over three hours. "Thank God," she reflected, "she pulled Lucas out with those things." Let's just say she appreciated her Chicago obstetrician's swagger.

Cesareans hold a similar place for some doctors. My colleague Stella, a maternal-fetal specialist, reflected that "after twelve years in midwifery practice before I went to medical school, I'm now so glad—so grateful—that I have the capacity to do a cesarean to save either the mother or the baby, when it's necessary." When she was a midwife, it was unnerving to think that cesarean wasn't a tool she had under her belt—that to save a life, she might have to ask someone for help.

Midwives have their own ways of dealing with birth's caprices. Some will insist on the trustworthiness of the body, on the normalcy of birth—which I think, perhaps having seen too much, is wishful thinking. Others, however, take care not to turn away from the unsettling facts of birth, but manage them with level heads and open dialogue about risk. But the nuance is lost in the acrimony of the birth wars. The continued insistence in books and blogs on the safety of birth and impropriety of technology reflects similarly an effort toward control, an effort to keep the unthinkable at bay and assure women, potential patients, that childbirth is invariably manageable the way midwives propose to effect it.

It is worth noting that, in no small part because of medical intervention and technology (antibiotics and safe cesarean, for example), birth is a considerably safer endeavor—at least in developed countries—than it was a hundred years ago. For instance, the number of deaths from maternity-related causes was approximately sixty-five times greater in 1900 than it was in the 1980s. At the turn of the twentieth century, about one woman would die for every 154 births recorded in the United States; if we take birth rates into account, this translates to one in thirty women who could have been expected to die in childbirth over the course of her fertile years. Infants fared worse; about one out of every eight babies died during delivery or within the first year of life. Advances in medicine, pediatrics, and maternity care have improved matters dramatically. But as historian Judith Walzer Leavitt has offered, the actual numbers may not correlate so neatly with our stance: "Whether dangers are reported as one in every 150 births or one in 10,000, women find themselves thinking about death as soon as they become pregnant." In listening to women, I can assure you this continues to be the case for many more than you'd imagine. It emerges for attendants too, control being one of the ways that we operate in its shadow.

Tess, one of the midwives we interviewed, reflected that control is an issue for any "attendant"—whether midwife or physician. "Midwives are really controlling people," she told us candidly. "Whether they think it or not, they like it to be a certain way. Just like some physicians like you to be in stirrups with your legs wide open, bed broken apart, there are some midwives who want to have you in a particular position or want to have you not in a particular place." Karen, a midwife who attends home births, told us she has her clients sign a consent form in which they agree to trust her judgment—that they can have freedom to the degree she thinks what they are doing is safe.

Bottom line, control is an issue for all of us: doctors, midwives, and parents alike.

The reasons *why* control matters so much has to do not just with questions of power and gender, but with the fact that, in addition to joy, birth brings us close to things that give us pause, that can unsettle us. This is true for expectant parents, and it is also true for their care providers.

For one, birth reminds us that there was a time when we didn't exist—it serves as evidence of finitude. What we usually notice of birth is what is there (a baby) rather than what once was unimaginably not. And yet the bigger questions reside with us too. I remember one afternoon in San Diego, where I'd just given a lecture and had stolen away from the conference to have lunch with my mom and my then six-year-old son, Charlie. We had a table looking out across the bay, which inspired my mom to share recollections of seeing that sparkling vista as a child. Then Charlie—French fry in hand but always listening—asked me, "Where was I then, Mom?" And I answered in the only way I knew how: "You were just a twinkle, honey." Not even in his father's eye. My husband, Kim, wasn't born yet either. Birth can remind us that there was a time before we were born, before our babies were born; just as it gives us hope, it bumps up against the fact of nonexistence. It is something that is hard—at best—to imagine.

People say they go into obstetrics because it is a "happy" field—and indeed it is, for the most part. But part of what makes a birth "happy" rather than just ordinary is that birth is an answer to the things we don't want to think about or can't imagine: infertility, loss, death. We are both joyful and relieved to hear of a healthy birth. The eloquent surgeon Sherwin Nuland has written that medicine "attracts people with high personal anxieties about dying" and that we "become doctors because our ability to cure gives us power over the death of which we are so afraid." But the emergence of a child does something similar, for parents and providers alike: it gives us hope, appears as an answer to the meaninglessness and emptiness that death evokes.

The women of the Good Birth Project brought up the relationship between birth and death time and again. Birth was often a salve, a source of hope or meaning, as it was for mother of three Carley in her most recent delivery. She told us that two months after she'd gotten pregnant, her husband's sister had tragically died. "The whole time we were saying to ourselves, if [his sister] has anything to do with it, we'll have a girl. But you really don't know." At the moment of birth—and blur of blood and the umbilical cord—she and Jim thought they'd had their third boy. But looking again, they realized they'd had a daughter, and went from simply joyful to awestruck.

"[Jim] felt like his sister was . . . in the room with us," Carley told us as we passed her the tissues. "He called his family, it was very emotional. I remember holding [our daughter], and being in awe."

Obstetricians and midwives are similarly buoyed by births—not just by the births of our own children, but by births we attend. It is perhaps obvious how this might be the case for Stella, whose patients are women with extremely complicated and risky pregnancies, who brush closely with death but for Stella's competent and high-tech care. She told me, "The whole opportunity to try to improve the outcome of pregnancy is what's exciting to me and what I feel my mission is in life."

But birth has a similar effect in the context of decidedly low-tech, low-risk births. Midwife Donna linked birth and death closely when reflecting tearfully on her early experiences in practice.

> I remember in the little hospitals where I worked in Kentucky and West Virginia, we always laughed; for every person who died that day, a new baby would come, actually about within an hour. Yeah. It would be just about somewhere in that hour's time, that somebody had just passed on, that you'd be running down the hallway to help a new baby come.

So you see, there are at least some of us for whom attending births provides affirmation of the variety Nuland describes; just like curing a patient, catching a baby gives us "power over the death of which we are so afraid." It is no wonder there are "birth junkies" willing to stay up nights into their sixties catching baby after baby.

To the extent that we practitioners interface with birth—not just that we help ensure its safe accomplishment but have some sort of existential reliance on it—it is no wonder that we feel the need to control it, to manage it, to take credit for it even. It is no wonder that we doctors feel we need to trace the fetal heart rate over the course of labor, even though the external monitors that are strapped to every laboring woman's belly don't improve the likelihood of healthy delivery in uncomplicated pregnancies, and even though they increase cesarean rates. It is no wonder that some doctors bristle when women come in with birth plans detailing things they'll refuse, a steely resolve to resist an intravenous line, a request or demand for intermittent monitoring. As noted obstetrician Michael Green once told *New York Times* reporter Denise Grady, taking the fetal heart monitor away from doctors would be "like ruthlessly yanking Linus's blanket away from him." Yes, we are trained to act on "abnormal" heart rate tracings, but the best studies show that just listening, intermittently, to the fetal heart rate is as effective in preventing death of the baby around delivery, admission to neonatal intensive care, low Apgar scores, and cerebral palsy as watching constantly the peaks and valleys that the pervasive technology produces. In truth, watching a fetal heart tracing is a source of comfort upon which we rely; it is what makes us feel safe and secure, that everything will be okay. Without it, we feel we are powerless against the enemy—loss, death, nonexistence. To take the monitor away would make some of us feel, in short, out of control.

Much has been made in the past couple of years of the human tendency toward "magical thinking," which psychologists tell us is a natural response to uncertainty and the unimaginable. There are things we do—cross fingers, knock on wood, continue on with irrational beliefs and behaviors—that, they argue, are a consequence of believing we can have more control over the world than we actually do, that there is a way to eliminate randomness, eliminate the possibility of things we dread. There seems to be plenty of magical thinking around birth: the way we doctors cling to the monitor and other technologies that lack evidence of benefit; the way others insist that birth is "normal" or "safe." Whatever its source, practitioners' need for control can bump up against a woman's need for it; imposition as such can be just as much a threat to the good birth as the uncertainties of physiology, fate, and all else that determines how a birth happens.

What to make of this need for control that we all feel around birth? First, it's important to understand that it's there when you talk to your doctor or midwife or read books or blogs advocating one approach to birth or the other, pressing readers to either side of birth debates, or when you help someone you love sift through their options. You need to know what's happening, what's at stake when a doctor or midwife seems controlling, perhaps overly so. Or even when they seem to promise beyond reason. All of us will try to provide certainty through our own worldview, through an approach we have ourselves settled on (or clung to) as responsible when it comes to attending birth. We practitioners, however diverse, are working against the same thing (loss, meaninglessness), and belief in one particular way of doing things can make us feel safe, or safer—and in control.

Second, if you are approaching birth, know that control need not be a chafe point, a source of tension between you and your doctor or midwife. Part of the trick is finding a good fit. I will tell you that for the birth of William (my fourth), I wanted someone to have a strong hand on the reins, to exert some control—to tell me to slow my life down, to make me stand on a scale, to remind me that I needed to take care of myself, to treat me like a patient and not just a friend, to be my doctor, to beat back *for me* the things I feared, to share substantively in the responsibility that was bringing a child into the world. I was busy and knew I was prone to jettisoning self-care, even when pregnant. I needed and wanted someone with a heavier hand. So I chose a doctor who I knew had one, who checked every box that either of us could conceive of, who wasn't afraid of telling (respectfully, mind you) an empowered woman what to do. Her style wouldn't appeal to everyone, but it is hard to get an appointment with her—she is breathtakingly popular.

If what I wanted doesn't appeal to you—and I accept that it may well not—there are other doctors and midwives who will stand farther to one side. Indeed, I had different needs in earlier births, and chose people who were fairly traditional in their approach, if considerably less controlling, and were at points more like good girlfriends than doctors. That might appeal to you. Or you might gravitate toward a general obstetrician, family practitioner, or midwife who pushes back against hospital routine and clears the way for more choice and control for patients than has been the norm; someone who provides gentler guidance than the doctors I've chosen for myself; for whom control is found in a different balance between trust and wariness of birth. Or you might choose someone like midwife Karen—who is likewise breathtakingly popular among women opting for home birth. She tells new clients that giving birth at home entails "a lot of responsibility" on their part because they are pulling away from standard practice. As such, she explains, they'll need to choose for themselves which offerings of modern medicine they will accept and which they will reject.

Now, I know I had an unfair advantage when it came to choosing a provider. I had a choice, for starters, and not everyone does—far from it. Often the way that medicine is organized means women have to take whom they get. In addition, the providers among whom I'd had the opportunity to choose I'd stood across from in an operating room; I knew how skillfully and under what circumstances they moved a scalpel, knew how they made decisions when pressed to the wall, knew how they reacted to birth. But if you do have a say in the matter, know that finding the right provider is not an exact science, and given the uncertainties of birth, whomever you choose may or may not end up being there to help usher you through. (Indeed, when I labored a day before one of my "scheduled" cesareans, two of the four hands at the operating table, though competent, were not the ones I'd expected.)

Still, the women I interviewed emphasized (and I agree with them) that it's worth the time and effort to consider whom you want there if you have the chance to do so. It's important to remember that it's not just about the doctor or midwife, but how you relate to *each other*, about that particular space that you two might share. Some women find it helpful to interview potential providers, get a sense of the fit—of their approach to birth, their style, their relationship with technology, the ways in which they maintain the sense of control to which we all aspire. But these sorts of conversations can mislead, so it's important, too, to be attuned to how the relationship feels over the course of the pregnancy, to trust your intuition and stay open to making a change if your sense of the fit starts to unravel. And keep in mind that most providers practice in groups, within which you'll invariably have a favorite, who may or may not make it to your bedside for birth. Not to worry, though—as the stories in this book will continue to show, having things unfold exactly as planned or preferred isn't a recipe for a good birth either.

These anticipatory conversations don't have to be exhaustive; a question or two can tell you a lot about a person's style. Take the varying approaches to weight gain in pregnancy. Do you want someone who will cite the guidelines that mark excess gain at thirty-five pounds and who will make sure you don't "overdo" it? Or do want someone who will tell you she has been there—pregnant and hungry—gained more, and that the weight will come off with some effort? Without even directly "interviewing," you can get a sense, in the first couple of appointments, of how a provider thinks about medicine, risk, uncertainty, and then consider for yourself whether their approach reassures or unsettles you. For instance, my friend Jackie loved her OB, who was Dutch and so, she said, had a "more global perspective" on birth. Without condemning the medical profession, he could tell her where Americans were "overreaching" in his view—and again where they were not. She didn't always agree, but liked how easily he shared with her his balanced skepticism. Not surprisingly, he also was open (even encouraging) of that occasional half glass of wine when she wanted it—no ban on toasting an anniversary with a bit of bubbly—despite the profession's official stance against even a sip. Even here, the point is not to micromanage a plan for birth, but to find someone with whom you feel comfortable, trust as a partner, and who can advocate for you when the unexpected hits.

At the end of the day—for those with some semblance of choice among providers, those without a choice at the outset, or those in delivery who are faced with a stranger from a large group practice rather than the reassuring visage of a person who has guided them through prenatal care—the themes that follow that emerged in the Good Birth Project will help you articulate what you need and advocate for yourself or someone you love, whoever it is that makes it to the bedside for delivery.

As you sift through your options, know that ultimately birth presses everyone up against the edge of life. We practitioners all have our own way of bearing witness, or not, to finitude; control is the means through which we do it. Appreciating that has helped me understand why doctors, midwives, and loved ones act the way they do, and figure out whom I want around me when giving birth myself. I hope it will help you too.

Finding Control, Finding "Good": The Things That Really Matter

It turns out that the women of the Good Birth Project really wanted something specific—something particular—when they said they wanted "control" in birth. My team and I listened for how women spoke about control, and what they meant when they used the term. We discovered that what women said they needed, even if its particularity ranged considerably, fell into five general categories, which comprise the next five chapters of this book.

For some women, control meant having a say in how birth unfolded. It meant being able to make decisions, feel that they were consulted and that their births were theirs, that they were able to bear witness—that birth wasn't "taken away from them." It related to the sense that they were involved—indeed, that they were giving birth rather than being delivered. I call this *agency*.

For others, control related to feelings of physical or emotional safety. Sometimes that derived from what was happening outside them—feeling like things around them were in order, not chaotic or "out of control." Sometimes it related to what was inside—whether they felt anxious or scared. I call this *personal security*.

Still others linked control with how connected they felt to other people. Feeling alone or isolated meant they were out of control. Feeling accompanied by a loved one or other support person or having trust in caregivers made them feel in control. I call this *connectedness*.

For other women, control related to what people often call "dignity" or "self-respect." Being in control meant being composed and calm on the outside, or feeling that they had mental strength and didn't let themselves "get in the way." This is a piece of what I came to call *respect*.

Other women said that information was integral to the sort of control that made birth good. They wanted to feel prepared, know what was going on, understand what was happening to their bodies. I call this *knowledge*.

Interestingly enough, even women who didn't use the term *control* understood the good birth as a function of one or more of the above. Liz may have used the word *control* in describing what was missing from her birth—when she was surrounded by strangers, unable to see her husband, worried about her baby's health—but others just talked about feeling afraid or abandoned. Control is a marker for the good in birth, but different people call it different things. Hence, this book is called *A Good Birth* and not *A Controlled Birth*. Control is tricky for a different reason as well: it can take a while to get a handle on the sort of control to which we should hold fast, versus the sort of control we need to release.

Maisie, twenty-seven, talked a lot about control—how she zeroed in on it over time. She had felt unnerved by her hospital births, and experienced hospital routines as oppressive, constraining. So she chose to have her third child at home because of the control it would give her over her surroundings, regardless of whatever her body was doing and however she was responding to the experience of birth. "It's funny," she said, "you could be in control of being out of control." For Maisie, control in birth stemmed from the freedom to do what she wanted to do, having her needs met, being treated with care and respect, and being able to focus on giving—and celebrating—birth. This was a kind of control that freed her to be "out of control": to sink into and relish birth in all its uncertainty and power.

To the degree that birth exceeds control—that we can be consumed by birth, overtaken by it, even ended by it—forging a good experience requires holding the incomprehensible at bay, maintaining a sense of self, and making meaning in the process. Having a birth in which what we need and value is honored will bring us closer to what I'll refer to as Maisie's Paradox: "in control of being out of control." Birth can be a moment full of uncertainty and chaos; with the birth of a child, specific plans will elude us, but with good care and attention to what is essentially at stake in birth, we can get what we need—the good birth will be ours.

In the next five chapters, I'll explore in turn the five factors women say are important to a good birth. How important each is will depend on the woman, her life circumstances, and her values. For any given woman, the relative importance of the five factors may change from one birth to the next. One or more may have particular resonance for you. As you consider them, remember that a good birth is not about checking boxes or acing all five. It is about shifting the conversation, orienting our choices about and assessments of birth around the things that mothers, wise women, say matter most.

two

Agency

I had to figure out how to push hard enough and get the baby out on my own. I had strong support . . . but . . . no one was going to deliver me of or from anything.

—FAULKNER FOX

But who gives it? And to whom is it given? Certainly it doesn't feel like giving, which implies a flow, a gentle handing over, no coercion . . . No one ever says giving death, although they are in some ways the same, events, not things. And delivering, the act the doctor is generally believed to perform: who delivers what? Is it the mother who is delivered, like a prisoner being released? Surely not; nor is the child delivered to the mother like a letter through a slot. How can you be both the sender and the receiver at once? Was someone in bondage, is someone made free?

—MARGARET ATWOOD

"I never told you," Susan said to me, "but I had two home births."

I can't say why she had felt like she needed to keep it a secret, like I wouldn't approve or something, being a doctor. I'd hired Susan five years before to help me pick out some drapes for our living room and transform it from its unruly kid-chaos to a place that adults might feel like having an adult conversation, might just feel like sitting down for a moment. And I'd say we became friends in the process—shared plenty about ourselves over swatches. Of course, maybe it just hadn't come up; she didn't know about my cesareans either. So I suppose we were even in keeping that part of ourselves to ourselves.

But when I told her I was writing a book about birth, she pulled me aside to talk about it. "It was thirty-five years ago," she reflected, "when doctors wouldn't budge. I wanted to do things my way, and I knew they wouldn't give me any choices in the hospital. They had their routines, you know, and they were resistant to change."

She didn't really want a home birth, she told me. What she wanted was a hand in the matter, the opportunity to make it her own. She didn't want to just conform to her doctor's plan. "Sure, some pain medicine would have been nice," she reflected, "but I was willing to trade pain for freedom."

Susan held fast to the notion that having options, being able to make choices, and shaping birth to the degree that it's possible are absolutely critical to its being a good experience. And the women of the Good Birth Project told us the same thing time and again. "Birth isn't something that just happens to you," reflected mother of three Carmen. "You do it." Or at least—the thinking goes—you should.

Understanding Agency

And so we come to the first of the five major elements of a good birth: something I've come to call *agency*. It's a word sociologists and philosophers use to describe the capacity of a person to act in the world, to make his or her own choices (as opposed to being someone to whom things happen). The idea is that a good birth is one that we have a hand in shaping—a birth that's informed by the things we value, a birth in which we've been able to decide among options, a birth in which we feel involved and present.

Agency requires we stand on that slippery edge of control—it's about having choices in the process of navigating something that no one really has the power to orchestrate. We need options, the opportunity to decide between them, and an actual experience of birth in which we feel engaged, a central actor, the author.

But how to understand agency in birth? Among the metaphors I've heard used to describe birth, there is at least one—the marathon—that I worry misleads us in our quest for agency. All too often I find that it gives the false impression that "success" can be found in the strong body and mind, in preparation and perseverance. It implies control in a sense that will elude us. This is not to say that birth is or should be considered a passive endeavor, something done to us rather than something we do. But for most women, the image of an open road imposes sentimental fantasies on birth, makes it seem like preparation and sheer force of will is what it takes to cross the finish line standing.

I like metaphors, though, and there is one that I think connotes more accurately the notion of agency to which wise women aspire. I'd say birth is much more like a channel crossing, a journey across a moving body of water. There are things we cannot control—the width of the crossing, the current, the winds, or the weather. Our choices will be bounded by necessity—sometimes a paddle will suffice; other times we may need a motor or help from a friend. The outcome will be shaped to some degree by luck, and it will not always be graceful. Part of the joy will come from the fact that when we arrive on the other shore, we can look back and know that the journey is behind us. But part of the joy will come from feeling that we have been at the helm, that we are not merely passengers, and that the journey has been ours.

The question, then, is how to make it so. In this chapter, I cover what have emerged in conversations with childbearing women as the building blocks of agency in birth: choice among options, being the deliverer—whether one is pushing a baby out or having a cesarean—and presence or being in the moment. Together these things make us feel that in the journey that is birth, we have, in some substantive way, been leading the way.

Being the Decider: Options and Choices

At its most basic, women giving birth need to feel like they can say what happens to their body—again basic things, like who touches it and when. No doubt, not having had these most fundamental of choices is part of why women and more broadly feminists pushed back against mid-century hospital routines in birth, part of why Susan couldn't picture giving birth within hospital walls, part of why midwives like Kitty Ernst came out fighting and continue to do so. To the degree that rights to bodily dominion continue to be tested and contested in birth, we need to remember where we've been, and no doubt be alerted to and concerned about things that threaten these rights. But a good birth depends on not just the absence of violation. I'd offer that having those things in place makes birth simply tolerable. A good birth demands more.

In birth, there is no way for our body not to be breached. We are delivering a child who has resided within us into the outside world, and we want to shape how it happens. As such, we want to know, realistically, what our options are, and we want the opportunity to understand and meaningfully decide among them. The impulse to shape how things happen no doubt has resonance for anyone undergoing a major life transition, for anyone who might enter a hospital, for anyone considering becoming a parent—whether or not their bodies are so intimately involved. But in birth, choice as such takes on a particular urgency. Listening to women's stories gives a clue as to why.

I'll begin with Natalie, mother of two and "wise woman" in all the ways we imagined when we coined the term to describe women who'd been through birth. Natalie will tell you that she wasn't exactly "in control" when she delivered Emmie, her first. Emmie emerged at the end of a forty-hour labor, tugged out with a vacuum by a doctor Natalie had never met. Nevertheless, Natalie told us, the birth was good because she could make choices that allowed her to approach birth in a way that had meaning for her.

Natalie didn't strike me as a typical "natural birth" mom. When I first met her, she was within weeks of giving birth to her second baby—a boy she'd name Joshua. Natalie's straight black hair was trimmed into a stylish bob, her lips betrayed a touch of gloss, and a crisp white maternity shirt with a bit of lace on the bottom edge graced her belly. Betraying my early intuitions, for her first birth, Natalie told me, she had been determined to deliver without anesthesia.

For Natalie and her husband, Rob, getting pregnant with Emmie had been "a bit of a process." After a long couple of years of first giddy, then planned mid-cycle sex, and hundreds of dollars spent on home pregnancy tests (all negative), they consulted a well-regarded fertility doctor at the academic medical center where they went for medical care. The news they got was entirely unexpected, and devastating: a blood test indicated Natalie's ovaries would not be able to produce healthy eggs; Natalie would not be able to have her own biological children. The doctor suggested they pursue an egg donor or adoption.

At first, Natalie said, it was a "big loss," but she started doing some research on her own, and in the corner of a local bookstore she found hope in a book about Eastern medicine, herbs, acupuncture, and fertility. After a few sessions of acupuncture, she wound up pregnant, delighted.

If you had asked Natalie years before, she would have told you that she'd be more comfortable in a hospital with doctors and nurses and medical equipment surrounding her. But this was the same community that had told her she wouldn't be able to conceive. "I think I started feeling . . . empowered, in that I was capable of doing something the Western doctors said I couldn't do, and that I could do this on my own." Her decisions about the sort of birth she wanted simply followed: "I was in the state of feeling like I want to do this as naturally as possible—this is the way we conceived, this is the way I want to do it."

And she did it: labored thirty-six hours, pushed for four, and delivered a "gorgeous baby daughter" without any pain medicine or epidural. It was a good birth, and centrally because she'd done what she had set out to do—had "felt empowerment during the whole process" and felt that she was the one in charge of herself and her body, especially in the aftermath of being told that she wasn't and that her ovaries had already "failed."

When I first started practicing obstetrics, I regarded my patients' choices to eschew epidurals with a mixture of skepticism and curiosity. I worried that some felt obliged to at least try because the choice lined up with what "good mothers" would do—endure pain for their kids—which seemed oppressive. That birth was "natural" didn't settle it for me—it wasn't enough to answer why women would forgo pain medication for a famously painful process. Concerns about the safety of epidurals also failed to settle the question. People didn't opt out of an epidural for knee surgery, and nobody was writing with any sort of passion or purpose about the "hazards of epidurals" for anything other than childbirth. Despite an array of claims about their implications, the research shows that while they do increase the chances a delivery will involve forceps or a vacuum (so a reason, possibly, to avoid epidural: to lower the chances of an instrumental birth), they have no effect on the risk of cesarean section or the health of newborns. The research to date also shows that when it comes to the effective treatment of pain, they work better than the alternatives—whether IV medication or nontraditional alternatives, like immersion in water, acupuncture, or hypnosis.

Natalie's interview casts a different light on decisions about pain medicine and delivery. For her, eschewing the epidural wasn't about safety or about a view of birth and birth pain as natural or normal. Instead, for Natalie, it was about taking back the reins that were being tugged away. It was about giving birth in a way that felt meaningful *to her.*

I really appreciated that Natalie didn't romanticize her "natural" birth or take it as evidence that one way of giving birth was necessarily better, or that she was better, somehow, than anyone else. Indeed, she used an epidural in her next pregnancy and felt "smarter" for it (more on that later). Her approach was rather the final chapter of a very personal struggle against infertility, against the specter of loss, against the possibility that she would not give birth in her lifetime.

I've learned since my early days on labor wards that other women value the choice of not having an epidural for other reasons. Some women really want the opportunity to walk around, or sit on a birthing ball, or just move when they are laboring, and that pretty much goes out the window when you have an epidural in place. Epidurals constrain certain options and require as a matter of safety and—yes, protocol—that you have an IV in place, because epidurals can make your blood pressure drop, and when that happens you may need some IV fluid to get it back up where it needs to be. And there are myriad other reasons that you'll learn about over the course of this book.

But not everyone finds meaning—or empowerment—in the rejection of technology. Not everyone feels liberated when medical procedures feel out of reach. Such was the case for Christina, who had to fight her way to a cesarean for the birth of her second child.

Like Natalie, Christina also had a hard time getting pregnant with her now six-year-old daughter. After three cycles of in vitro fertilization, she conceived and had twelve embryos to spare, which her doctors froze in case she wanted to have another baby later. Entering birth, she didn't have a bone to pick with doctors or technology. "I'm in awe of technology," she told us. "I'm in awe and I'm grateful it was there for me."

She'd also considered a "natural" birth, but it was really about safety. "I thought, 'I don't want any chemicals entering the poor baby. Can the poor baby take this?'" Of course, one of the advantages of epidurals (over intravenous drugs) is that the pain medications stay put in the area around the spine and don't reach the bloodstream of mother or baby, so that wasn't in truth a worry about the epidural. So with contractions that felt excruciating, Christina ended up getting an epidural and was happy the option was available. "I'm going to use modern medicine where I can to help me," she said, laughing. "Why suffer?"

But Christina's first birth was scary, long, and complicated by shoulder dystocia (an obstetrical emergency in which a baby's shoulder gets stuck behind the mom's pelvic bone after the head delivers) and a cord wrapped three times around her daughter's neck. It was so scary that afterward Christina thought for a long time she'd have only one baby. She loved being a mom; she'd always wanted two children—wanted to give her daughter a sibling. But for Christina birth had been "traumatic" and she didn't want to do it again. She didn't want to replay the moment of terror when her baby came out looking "very dark" and not breathing or crying, didn't want to endure the recovery, and didn't want another spate of painful memories.

She thought about adopting, but something else tugged at her. "I had those embryos," she said, "and I couldn't leave them." So eventually she used them. Pregnant at forty-five, she was hopeful she could persuade a doctor to go straight to a cesarean. Given that she'd delivered vaginally and didn't have a "medical" indication for an elective cesarean (having been terrified didn't count, though a prior dystocia might have), it was a hard sell, but she was relentless in her request, and eventually her doctors agreed.

I imagine I would have agreed too. Listening to Christina, her request seemed utterly reasonable. She didn't see any magic or meaning in vaginal birth: she wanted a delivery that was contained and predictable—and nobody could convince her that vaginal birth would be either of these things. She understood that cesarean delivery was "major surgery" and "not to be taken lightly." But the latter, she'd concluded, was also true of vaginal birth. "Knock me out and take it out, please," she remembered thinking. "I can't do that again. It affected my life too much."

Some people might blame the events that terrified Christina on the epidural—or doctors, or the hospital, or Christina's sense during her first pregnancy that her body was somehow dysfunctional because she'd needed medical help to conceive. Indeed, some women like Christina might find solace in distance from the hospital, or in new relationships and the new faces and philosophies they entail. For Christina, though, the promise of a "gentle birth" fell flat; rather, access to surgery and its certainties was her new notion of a "good birth."

Christina wasn't disappointed. She ended up delivering her son at term by cesarean, and told us she was glad for the choice, glad the decision was ultimately hers. Comparing her two deliveries, she said they were "like night and day. [The cesarean] was a great experience. I'm glad I had the choice."

Natalie and Christina had very different experiences, and both would tell you they valued them, that they felt they had "good births." Both women had a hand in how things unfolded, and both were allowed to give birth in a way that had meaning for and made sense to them.

It's not just about major choices either. Many women say that they found what they needed in smaller things. Like mother of six Jen, who gave birth four times in a hospital and twice at home, and told us that the more mundane choices were what mattered to her.

> The feeling of being out of control, for me, is unavoidable. If there are any other things that I can control, like not leaving for the hospital, or eating pizza, then I think that kind of thing boosts my confidence enough that I feel like, okay, I can do this—I know there are going to be moments when it's going to be bad and going to be painful, but there are still these things that I can control.

For my friend Rachel, who gave birth three times by cesarean, there was just one choice upon which her good birth depended. Even with all the uncertainty surrounding her births, what made them good, she told me, was feeling like there was some part of the birth that she owned, that she could direct. She recognized it immediately after her most recent delivery when the neonatologists wanted to take her newborn to the nursery, monitor the baby's blood sugar, and perhaps give her a bit of formula. "It was then that I lost it. If they'd taken her, that birth would have gone from good to horrible. What went into my baby's body was the only thing I felt like I could control, and they were going to take it away from me."

One problem that comes up is that some choices are deemed more reasonable, more "respectable" than others. Christina bumped up against this when her reason for *requesting* a cesarean wasn't on the usual list of "indications." Some women, on the other hand, will face it in their *refusals* of interventions that are part of a hospital routine.

There is resistance by a considerable swath of patients to having an IV, for instance. From my standpoint as an obstetrician, the IV had never struck me as a big deal—a needle in the arm, just in case. It didn't seem invasive in the same way that surgery or a vaginal exam or an epidural can be. And it could be lifesaving. Having been tasked under duress with placing an IV in a hemorrhaging patient's arm a time or two made the decision to delay it seem unwise at best. Why not place it, I thought, when all was calm rather than when it was urgently needed, in the midst of an emergency?

It strikes me now that at least for some women the IV is akin to postnatal feeding (*à la* Rachel), pizza (*à la* Jen), or anesthesia-free birth (*à la* Natalie). For some women being able to decide how and when their body can be breached by a needle, whether their veins should be open to salt water, feels like something worth fighting for. As we've already discussed in this chapter, birth can feel like a challenge to bodily dominion, and I can see how the IV could be conceived as a last bastion of control. I can't say I've ever recommended delaying an IV—or even offered placement or not, proactively, as a choice between reasonably equal options. But I have come to understand women's resistance to IVs and respect their informed choices to eschew them in labor.

This is one of the things that tends to draw women toward midwives— their emphasis on and respect for women's choices. No doubt if you deliver outside a hospital, you won't have to say no as often if things like IV fluid and monitors feel invasive and you want to avoid them. For instance, Alex, who delivered three times at a freestanding birth center, liked how that approach allowed for "more flexibility. That's what I wanted. The ability to have choices and make decisions, because I don't want to just be told what to do and lay down and have a baby."

But out-of-hospital birth also will exclude options—epidurals and oftentimes pharmacologic pain medication being two of them. If you value these things, the hospital may strike you as a more "flexible" environment, because the things you value are there. Lainey, for instance, wanted pain medicine in labor and found its provision—in the hospital—imparted a sense of control.

> I got to say when I wanted pain meds and when I didn't. And I had a little button I could push to give myself more of the epidural, and I pushed that sucker a lot during the pushing. That gave me a feeling of control. I didn't have nurses saying, "Here, take these drugs and don't ask why." I felt like [my husband] and I and [the midwife] and our nurse were all working together and that I was an active participant. I mean, that's kind of obvious— I was the one pushing—but I just felt so incredibly involved and in control.

Part of this is about being able to make choices. In birth (no less than in life), our choices are bounded—there are things we can't control with certainty: when or how we labor; how it feels; how large our baby is and how we are shaped, inside; how people around us act, to name a few. But there are decisions to be made, and the freedom to choose between options is key to conceiving our births as good.

Being the Deliverer: Giving Birth

> *It makes me sad when women have had a cesarean and feel like they've failed . . . They have birthed their child in whatever way, they have helped bring new life into the world, and what a gift—it's a miracle every time. And I think most women are able to appreciate that. When they're able to step back and glory in their beautiful baby, and they recognize the miracle that their child is, and they're able to accept their part in that and glow from that. And I hope that's true many more times than it is not.*

> —STELLA, OBSTETRICIAN

Lainey's reflections bring up a second point. What she appreciated was not just that she got to make choices but that she was "involved." At first glance, this seems like a strange thing to say. Of course, any woman having a baby is involved; it can't happen without her. But there is something different about having a baby from, say, getting an appendectomy. While it's important that doctors ask our permission for any medical intervention, few people want to be "an active participant in" surgery to remove an inflamed organ or fix a bum knee. Bringing a baby into the world is a different situation entirely. To that end, being "the deliver*er*" pertains to how we talk and think about a woman's role in the birthing process; and it's about treating the birthing woman as the star of the show.

"I know this sounds bizarre," reflected midwife Bev, when we asked her what makes for a good birth, "but it's really true. I try to make women a part of it. It's like saying, 'This is your experience. And we are going to help you, because we can see what's going on—how to push a little better or get in a good position, but this is your experience, this is your baby.'"

This is not a new idea, and it is part and parcel of midwifery's approach to birth. The point was made in the early 1980s by sociologist Barbara Katz Rothman, who wrote, "When the *doctor* is delivering the baby, the mother is in the passive position of *being delivered*." Midwives have long recognized the offense of such language and refer to themselves as "baby catchers" to emphasize their sensitivity to this point. Even pediatrics guru Dr. Sears gives a nod to this in his *Baby Book* when he recounts attending the birth of his sixth child. "When I boast to friends that I delivered our baby, [my wife] Martha is quick to correct me. She delivered Matthew, I caught. Why should dad get all the credit when mom did all the work? Martha is right."

We in obstetrics still make the mistake; we say we deliver babies, but we don't, really. We catch them too, and tug them out sometimes. But the agent in the process is the woman. She is the one who gives birth—who gestates the child, labors, and delivers, vaginally or by cesarean. She does the real work of birth. She becomes the mother.

Confusion about this is not limited to hospital wards. People I love very much—like my mom—will talk about how many babies I've delivered, referring to the hundreds of patients' births I've attended and often recounted when she was willing to lend an ear. But when asked for the number by a friend or patient, I always say, "Four. I've delivered four beautiful boys." People puzzle at that, especially those who know how many years I practiced, how much of my thirties were spent on the hallways of Labor and Delivery, how many soiled pairs of clogs I've retired. And when I feel up to explaining, I give them the rest, the lesson I learned from midwives and agree with wholeheartedly: "Oh, yes. I've attended hundreds of births. But obstetricians don't deliver babies, women do."

This is not hair-splitting. That someone else could be given credit for the birth of my four children, and I for only the hundreds other than my own, seems ludicrous—right? But it reflects a long-standing tussle, and as a source of confusion it is remarkably entrenched.

About a month ago, I was reviewing an article for a scientific journal when I came across the word *accoucheur*. My college French has disintegrated considerably and it wasn't a term my obstetrical colleagues used much. The article reported a study about different approaches to clamping the umbilical cord and compared births where the *accoucheur* cut the cord to those in which it was cut by an assistant.

My initial recollection was that the verb *accoucher* had something to do with lying down, but I couldn't imagine that women themselves were doing the cutting, so I made my way to the dictionary. What I found was that *accoucheur* sits right on the debated edge of agency. As a verb, *accoucher* means "to be in labor, to give birth," but as a noun *accoucheur* describes not the childbearing woman but the care provider, specifically the "male obstetrician or midwife." Its origin dates back to the 1750s, so clearly who it is that gives birth has been an enduring source of confusion.

Semantics like this matter because language matters to women. Words uttered in deliveries get chiseled into our memories of the day; they shape our sense of what we did or didn't do. And part of a good birth is feeling like you did it, like it was *you* who brought the baby into the world.

Consider mother of four Olivia, who gave birth across the gamut of possible places (hospital, birthing center, and home)—so fiercely independent that she decided the fourth time around to give birth without assistance. No doubt she was sensitive to the question of who "does" birth and recalled for us a moment in her birth-center birth that still niggles her, which made it less than good.

A couple times [the midwife] said some things with kind of an attitude that made me think that she was like, "Just lie down, let me birth this baby." She didn't say that exactly, but that was kind of the attitude behind it, which was really different than how she acted the rest of the time.

But those of us who appreciate with equal conviction the need for assistance in birth also want to feel like (and be acknowledged as) the deliverer. This came through in mother of two Sharon's reflections about her first birth. She'd wanted to "go natural," but at thirty-six weeks her water broke and she developed signs of a uterine infection. Her doctor recommended that they give her some Pitocin, a medicine to hasten delivery. She labored quickly and delivered her six-pound daughter vaginally into the hands of a nurse, the doctor on call still drying off from a stolen shower. He arrived in time to treat Sharon for a massive postpartum hemorrhage, which required a trip to the operating room to contain.

Sharon insisted that the chaos of delivery and postpartum drama didn't detract. "I had a good birth," Sharon reflected. "You know, I really did. I felt like *I contributed to it*. I could feel my daughter coming, and I pushed her out."

But not everyone gets to push their baby out the way Sharon did. Some babies must also be pulled out with a vacuum or forceps (often while a woman pushes), and some will exit through their mother's belly wall, making the notion of doctors doing the delivering seem, if somewhat obnoxious, more to the point—an accurate account of what has happened during the course of delivery. So what to do when this happens—when medicine's instruments or interventions are required?

The first thing to realize is that birthing is birthing, however you do it. Some women need more help than others, but there isn't one kind of birth that "counts" and another that somehow doesn't. Going back to that channel-crossing metaphor, sometimes you need just a paddle, and sometimes you need a motor.

But what about cesareans? In what possible sense are women the ones who deliver the baby when the surgeon is the one making an incision, cutting through the uterine wall, pulling out the child? I understand the press, having experienced four such surgeries, four births, as a patient and mother.

Indeed, there is a sense that certain ways of birthing count more. Colleen, who chose to deliver by cesarean for her first birth, put it this way:

> I do get asked that question a lot, like, "Don't you want to experience the birth experience?" And I say, "I have experienced the birth experience, it's just different than yours." And I don't think people understand that. They're like, "Don't you want a *real* delivery?" And I'm like, "It is a *real* delivery." See, to me, I don't think that I needed to push her out the birth canal in order for it to be considered any more meaningful to me, so . . . but I do get that. I don't feel like I missed out on anything. Maybe some pain and anxiety.

What Colleen knows well is that there is more than one way to feel like you've done something extraordinary in birthing a child. Many women, whatever their delivery mode, felt proud of what they'd accomplished, as they should.

But it can take some reorienting because too many people presume that birth is defined by what happens the moment a child is born, and it's simply not. The women of the Good Birth Project remind us that the act of pulling (or pushing) the baby out is not the whole of birth. No doubt it's a moment fetishized, imagined as representative of the experience. But when we asked women to define "the birth experience," they talked about much more. Some said it started when they walked into the hospital, others when they felt the first contraction, and still others when they found out they were pregnant. A few even said birth started when they decided they wanted a baby, before the child was even conceived. There was similar breadth on the far end of birth: some said it was over when their child was in arms, or at home with them. Some said it ended weeks or months after delivery, and one in ten told us that "it never ends." Not a single woman said birth begins with the emergence of a baby's head or ends with the emergence of her feet.

The point is: To presume that agency—"birthing," as such—turns on the moment or mode of birth, on whether your child was born vaginally or by cesarean, misses the point, misses the fact that birth is a *process* that includes the purposeful and creative work of gestation, labor, delivery, and their aftermath.

The other thing women tell us is that pushing a baby out of one's body isn't the only way to feel involved—to feel a part of birth—even in the moment our children emerge. Mother of four Raquel told us that of all her births, she thought her last—and her only cesarean—was "every bit as positive as any of my other deliveries, if not my best delivery." Even though she was numb from the waist down, it's clear from listening to her that she felt very much a part of the project and process of birthing. The moments she recalled for us aren't the usual ones you might associate with empowered birth. Rather than holding her leg, her husband was holding a camera, but still encouraging Raquel, sharing with her what his vantage point offered, telling her she was doing a great job. Rather than work through contractions, she held fast while an epidural was placed and then while the tiny obstetrician on call helped her deliver by pouncing as we often do on her belly. Rather than talk with a doctor or midwife working between her legs, she joked with the surgeons whose faces she could see over the drape, one remarking he'd let his daughter date her baby someday, since he was so cute. I've been to deliveries like Raquel's—as both a doctor and a patient: full of joy and due regard for the mother who is giving birth. Indeed when William was born, even though someone else pulled him from my body, there was no question in my mind—or seemingly anyone else's in the operating room—that I was giving birth, that I did it.

A paper I love by philosopher Hilde Nelson makes the point about pregnancy, about the "work" of gestation that only women do. Drawing on Marx's distinction between the architect, who builds purposefully, and the bee, who "cannot help what she is doing," Nelson argues that human pregnancy is "in a number of respects purposeful, creative, and deliberate"—much more like the work of the thoughtful architect than the bee. Unlike other animals, we are often pregnant for a *reason*—because we want a baby, a sibling for our child, a family. Gestation involves *crafting a relationship*; the fetus we gestate becomes by virtue of our activity something we value, perhaps something we love. And in gestation, Nelson argues, we use our bodies to make a home—an activity she notes involves "far more than blind, uncomprehending nature." And finally we do our work—craft our house, so to speak—within the biological and social context that is life today. That might require figuring out how to manage the challenges of caring for a toddler and a growing belly at the same time, or making the decisions that come with medical conditions like depression or allergies during pregnancy, or continuing a job that requires balancing ambition and health. No doubt gestation is the expectant mother's work: we are active, we are the agent of birth no matter whether the hands that pull a baby from the body belong to us, to a trusted midwife or doctor, or even perhaps to someone we've never met. To imagine us as passive by virtue of person or mode is to forget the massive effort, the massive activity that birth as a whole entails.

Part of agency—part of feeling like the deliverer—is going to come from how you yourself see and understand birth, from taking to heart the corrective offered by Dr. Nelson and so many of the women we interviewed, from believing that nobody "does birth" but the childbearing woman herself.

But none of us lives in a vacuum, and it sure helps to have people around us acknowledge that we mothers are in fact the ones who give birth, who deliver. No doubt feelings of agency can be shaped by how people around us speak and act.

For those of you facing your own deliveries, I know, you're not in control of how people around you act. But emphatic shifts in the way you talk to those people can help (ask your doctor or midwife how many *deliveries she's attended*, not how many *babies she's delivered*). It may even help to be more explicit, to remind those around you who is doing the delivering (you); or that while the birth may be momentous for them (if they are your partner or parent, for example), you are the one giving birth, and on this day of days their focus needs to be on you. Indeed, for the partners, friends, and parents who support women in birth, acknowledging what a childbearing woman is doing or has done to bring a child into the world can be a powerful way to reinforce the sense of agency that is part of a good birth.

And it's an important lesson for midwives, doctors, and others who attend birth: we need to give credit where credit is due. A woman should never have to remind us that she has given birth, that *she* has delivered a baby. She has. We need to acknowledge what women do in birth and thank the women whose deliveries we attend for the honor of *helping* them bring a child into the world.

Indeed, the women of the Good Birth Project note the importance in birth of feeling not like just an active player, but like the *central* player in what feels like one of life's most important dramas. Alisa, a mother of five, recalled her good birth, noting, "I was treated so special, like, 'This is all about you and having your baby,' and nobody else in the world seemed to matter then." When reading through the interviews, we saw this theme often enough to dub it "Queen for the Day."

What Alisa says is key: women need to feel like "nobody else in the world seemed to matter." Most of the time, when we aren't giving birth, everyone else *does* matter: women have a tendency to put others' needs before their own—a tendency that motherhood only amplifies. Indeed, once the baby is born, the experience of being the central player in much of anything becomes a rarity for many women.

But in birth, we simply need to be the center, we need to be queen. And it's not just wanting a swan song for life as we know it, or getting credit where credit is due. It's also instrumental—it allows us to be fully focused on the task at hand. It takes different things for different women to feel like they are queens. Take my good friend Madeline, a kindergarten teacher, avid gardener, and busy mom. She relished her second birth for its fluffed pillows, heated blankets, and staff who were uniformly warm and attentive. Her birth was good, she told me, because she felt like she was "in a spa." Nobody ever fluffed pillows for Madeline unless she was somewhere that she could pay someone to do it (like a spa), but in birth she was the queen and got the special treatment she valued, deserved, and needed.

Megan also talked about the importance of this sort of queen treatment, how much she appreciated that she had the nurses' undivided attention leading up to her scheduled cesarean.

> They took me into an operating room, which was like a meat locker! It was freezing in there! [But] these nurses came and brought me these heated blankets—they were like rubbing my arms. I mean, that's the one thing I could say, is that *the nurses were totally focused on me* and, you know, "What can I do to make you feel better?"

Other women, conversely, recoiled at the recollection of their partner complaining that he hadn't eaten or that he was tired. What I'd like to offer here is that we should remind ourselves and others that it's not like we don't care. It's that we can't. Because birthing is one of life's most consuming tasks. It is not a time when we can attend to someone else's needs. If we think they'll come up and detract from our experience or our ability to focus, a doula or family member who understands the consuming nature of birthing can be incredibly helpful in keeping us and our needs center stage.

The bottom line is that women giving birth want and need the singular focus of those who attend them in birth. They need to know they are seen and heard, that they are understood to be the central actor in the unfolding drama of the day, that in the massive undertaking that is giving birth, they are the ones doing the birthing.

Presence

There is a third piece to agency as well. It is the need to be present, to "be there" for birth, to give birth "in awareness." The need for presence is something that I've noticed far and wide, in literature and history, across providers with divergent approaches to birth, across women of myriad backgrounds. All say that being present and aware holds a solemn, almost sacred importance.

You might wonder what being present for birth has to with agency. After all, all sorts of people can be present for a birth—medical students, family members, journalists, laboratory technicians—and have no agency whatsoever when it comes to the birth they witness, nothing to do with how that birth unfolds. Indeed, one version of presence leads us to imagine a spectator of birth, someone on the sidelines. Not someone who presides, but someone who watches, passively: applied to a childbearing woman, such is hardly the stuff of a good birth as I've portrayed it thus far.

But there is a decidedly active notion of presence that earned its place here in my chapter on agency. Of course, there are ways that presence is a *means* to agency in birth: you need to be "in the moment" if you are going to make decisions about your birth; and you also need to be "in the moment" if you are to conceive of yourself as the deliverer, the person doing the birthing. But presence also earns its keep as an end in itself. Because presence is not just about being there for birth; it is about *bearing witness* to it.

Bearing witness is not a passive endeavor—far from it. According to journalism professor Sue Tait, bearing witness "exceeds seeing"; rather, it is something that we *do*. For journalists it links observation with responsibility and serves to "immortalize events that are tied to the mortal bodies that go through them." According to the dictionary, to *bear witness* is "to show by your existence that something is true."

I am not sure whether either of these conceptions of bearing witness quite get to the heart of what presence means to childbearing women, or why it is that presence is so very important to them. What I am sure of, though, is that there is a deep and profound value to witnessing birth, being "there" for it, however it unfolds. Listening to women suggests that there is something pressing about witnessing birth, something critical and formative about it, something relevant to the agency that a good birth requires. Going back to our channel crossing, when you are standing on the other side, you need a sense of how you got there.

Indeed, when natural-birth convert Natalie looked back on Emmie's birth, she told me, there was something missing after all. Coupled with the sense that she had done what she had set out to do was the sense that she had missed something precious in the process of her daughter's birth. After four hours of pushing, her midwife suggested that Natalie probably needed help to get her baby's head past her prominent pelvic bone, and the midwife recommended a vacuum, a small suction cup that would be placed on the baby's head. Ultimately Natalie agreed, and with the entry of the pediatrics and obstetrics team into her room, the birth—her birth—became "someone else's" and the pain "unbearable."

> I was totally separate from the experience. I mean, it was totally its own thing, its own experience . . . The pain was bad, but it was something I had been managing. But then when the lights came on [and the doctors came in], it was a totally different story. And it was someone else's delivery almost . . . I just lost my

focus . . . It was kind of like I guess riding a bucking bronco, and like you're holding on, you're holding on, you're holding on and you're fine, and then all of a sudden I just totally lost it. And that was painful.

The bad part of her "good" birth, in essence, was that she missed it—as she describes it, she was "totally separate from the experience."

For her second birth, Natalie deliberated throughout her pregnancy—was still deliberating when I first met her—but ultimately chose to use an epidural. A good part of her reason was simply exhaustion: "I was really tired. And I didn't feel like fighting the fight of labor when I didn't have to. So towards the end, it was my body kind of naturally telling me, 'Give in to this one. If you can just sit and relax and watch TV while you're in labor, go ahead and do it.'"

What was surprising to Natalie, though, was that "giving in" also brought her what, later, struck her as missing from her first birth: not pain relief per se, but rather a chance to bear witness. As she explains:

Having [my mind] off the pain, I was able to focus on the rest of it. Be present. Really be present for [our son's] arrival. And I didn't feel present for [our daughter's]. And so that was fantastic . . . it was a really, really good experience, and not at all what I had expected.

Natalie's birth brings up an important lesson, which is that decisions about anesthesia are not just decisions about pain but about *presence*—about being in the moment, having access to the experience, capturing for oneself what birth is and what it means. If you think I'm making a plug for epidurals, I'm not. It's not about epidurals; it's not even about pain. It's about something that women across the Good Birth Project find to be important in birth—being present, aware, in the moment.

Certainly, Natalie wasn't alone in identifying the epidural as a helpful means to that end. Mother of two Kia recollected getting pressure from her own mother to eschew the epidural for her second birth, but she resisted, citing presence—wanting to "be there"—as the reason.

It's my birth experience—I'd rather be there than to feel so much pain that I don't want to be bothered with the baby when I deliver. Once I was given the epidural, I was able to relax a little better and focus on getting the baby delivered without having to worry about how much pain I am going through.

But other women find different ways to feel present. For some, like Serena, twenty-two, unanesthetized birth can get them the presence they value. For her first baby, Serena had endured an emergency cesarean for high blood pressure, during which her epidural wasn't working well, so she needed extra pain medicine via an IV to make it through. "They told me they put the baby to my face and said it was a boy, but I didn't see," she told us with an uncomfortable laugh, "because I was so drugged."

After that harrowing experience, delivering vaginally became something she desperately wanted to do, wanted to experience. Why? She wanted to be present, feel birth, see her baby emerge. Comparing her cesarean and vaginal births, she notes:

> The C-section is bad because you don't get to see your baby come out . . . During the vaginal delivery, you can feel everything, feel the contractions, feel the kicks, feel the movement, and you get to be awake for it the whole time. You get to see [the baby] come out, you get to feel it, you get to feel the afterbirth come out.

In contrast, mother of two Sally found in her cesarean the very presence Serena had noted was missing in hers. In her first birth, Sally had hoped to deliver in a local freestanding birth center. But after nearly thirty hours of labor, she transferred to the hospital fully dilated but exhausted, and she ended up with a cesarean. At the time, she notes, she was sorely disappointed in herself, in her body. Despite that, she described her son Travis's birth as good.

> But his actual birth—he was healthy, I was aware of him. You know, I would define that as a good birth. I didn't really feel like I wanted a mirror there to be watching even if he'd been born

vaginally. That wasn't important to me. But to be awake . . . was really important. So I was able to see him as soon as they pulled him out. They showed him to me, took him to the table that they cleaned him on and checked him out on right behind us.

In fact, presence was one of the reasons Colleen chose cesarean for her first birth. She didn't have a medical "indication" for surgical delivery but felt that it offered her what she valued in birth—a higher likelihood of presence being among the reasons she chose it. She explains:

One of my best friends had a delivery where she was in labor for almost forty-eight hours and ended up with a C-section, and was put to sleep and missed all of it. So I said, "Well, this way I'll be awake and get to see my baby as soon as we are all done." So I chose the elective cesarean for that.

Presence takes many forms. For some, like Serena, it's about bodily experience—it's about *feeling* birth. For others, like Natalie, Sally, and Colleen, it's more a cognitive experience—it's about seeing or witnessing the event. Parsing through wise women's reflections on presence, it turns out that their reasons for wanting or valuing it are as diverse as their birth stories. But I think it is safe to say that, for all of us, presence was an ingredient critical to making meaning of our births, savoring their sweetness, and sifting through the rest.

Take Sally again, for example. She hadn't wanted to deliver by cesarean, but her birth was still good. In fact, she told us she treasures it, and one moment in particular: the moment, mid-cesarean, when she learned the sex of her child.

She and her husband had decided not to find out beforehand; they wanted to be "surprised." But it was more than that. Sally told us her father had died just months before she got pregnant. Her grandmother—alive and well—had unthinkably lost a son, and said to Sally when she got pregnant, "God would not take away a boy and not give me a boy."

So waiting to find out the sex of her child had a certain seriousness to it, like waiting to open that letter that promises to seal a fate, shift a story. For many of us, finding the right moment to break such a seal makes all the difference, as it did for Sally. Mid-cesarean was that very moment: "I can tell you that when they said, 'It's a boy' [pause], I can't even describe how exciting it was. Like a hundred Christmases cannot add up to what an exciting event that was."

She named the baby after her father, first and middle names. "It was just a very nice cycle," she said. A reminder, indeed, that birth is, centrally, about ushering in a life, about the ways we humans cross the boundaries of existence. Bearing witness to that—whether in an operating room, a birthing room, or a home, is I think central to what a good birth is all about.

Clearly there are many ways to achieve presence, and it will mean different things to different people. Heading toward birth, it may seem elusive, since it's hard to tell how pain—or pain medicine—will affect you, and how your birth will go. But I do think focusing on presence clears the way for better decisions about pain medicine in a way that issues of safety or normalcy as goals do not. Despite the heated debates about pain management in birth, the fact is that anesthesia is safe *and* that a good birth does not depend on the absence of pain. Recently, the *American Journal of Obstetrics & Gynecology* published a major systematic review of the literature on pain and women's satisfaction with the experience of childbirth and concluded that "the influences of pain, pain relief, and intrapartum medical interventions on subsequent satisfaction are neither as obvious, nor as direct, nor as powerful as the influences of the attitudes and behaviors of caregivers." For some women, one conclusion might be that relief of pain is not necessary for satisfaction with the birth experience, so let's jettison the epidural and its attendant risks and downsides.

Presence pulls us away from the questions about the safety or usefulness of interventions for pain control and brings into focus what is beneath those questions and the discord that surrounds them—it helps us home in on what is essentially at issue for many of us when we give birth. To argue about epidural anesthesia as an end in itself—a "good" thing or a "bad" thing—misses the point. Pain and pain relief may both have a "purpose" in birth. The purpose of each, in fact, may be one and the same, depending on the woman, her situation, her health, and the circumstances surrounding her particular pregnancy. Either can be key to achieving *presence* in the experience of giving birth. If you are looking toward birth, considering these options for yourself, how to decide what is right for you?

Begin by casting aside those distracting (and flawed) notions that good mothers give birth naturally or sensible mothers give birth with the assistance of modern medicine. Think instead about presence when you are sifting through options. It may be a reason to eschew pain medicine altogether (Might your efforts to manage pain focus your mind? Whom do you need around you to make that possible?) or to use a technique, like hypnosis, that allows ready access to experience. Partners and loved ones can help some women cope with pain effectively and maintain a sense of presence. Or do you think pain itself, even with coping and other techniques, will be "distracting"—as it was for many of the women we interviewed? If you opt for anesthesia, remember that intravenous narcotics will make you loopy; epidurals won't. So even if epidurals seem more "invasive," they are considerably less likely to interfere with your feelings of presence and so might be preferable. Nitrous oxide (gas you breathe through a mask)—available in only a few centers in the United States but more widely across Europe—gets out of your system in minutes, so that if you start to feel alienated from your birth (read: too loopy) you can hang it up quickly. If you end up needing a cesarean, remind your anesthesiologist that you want to be awake and aware for the delivery. Tell him it matters to you that you're not sleepy, that you want to see it, you want to be there for it. And don't be afraid to talk to the surgeons—we're used to it. Remind them that you're there, and with any luck they'll treat you like you are.

And it's another lesson for providers: we all need to keep presence in mind, and be open and creative about ways to help childbearing women feel "in the moment." When indicated, we need to think about pain medicine or antiemetics that don't sedate. Whatever the mode of delivery, part of our job is to affirm, acknowledge, and facilitate a woman's sense that she is there; describe for her things she cannot see but wants to; help her bear witness to the birth of her child.

Again, I know this sounds strange, but many an operating room I've been in has a sign reminding obstetricians and others there that "the patient is awake." It's bizarre that any person attending birth would need a reminder, but many do, given that most of the time the (nonpregnant) people on whom doctors operate are asleep and want to be. If you are on the operating table, don't be afraid to make yourself known.

The other thing to remember is that there are ways to bear witness that don't rely on in-the-moment awareness. No doubt some women won't, for myriad reasons, get to witness their births in the moment and that can feel like a big loss. A few of the women we interviewed had to be asleep for their births, usually for serious medical reasons. Karla had a brain tumor, and Jill had a serious liver condition that almost took her life; many others were exhausted or nauseated or scared or had a reaction to medicine that cast a haze over the event. But, they told us, there were things that made a difference to them, that made them think about their births as good births, that made them feel more present: among these were photos, conversations with others who did see everything, and having someone else with them, observing, for whom the birth was similarly monumental.

Indeed, Jill wasn't just asleep for her good birth—after the cesarean she had to go to intensive care and stay asleep for a couple of days; some of the medicines they gave her wiped out her memories, even of times when she had been awake. But she told us how she recrafted the birth, pulled together the pieces she needed: photos of her holding her baby for the first time (which she didn't remember), recollections of her parents and husband, and her own first memory of laying eyes on her baby. And once she felt lucid, she told us, "I kind of went into my planning mode again. I got a legal pad and a pen and said [to the doctors], I want to know everything that has happened to [my baby] in the last week . . . So that was good—it helped kind of fill in the gaps." Jill told us that she is still a little frustrated about the wiped-out memories, but accepts they were necessary to her good birth, to her getting to the other side of the channel in one piece.

Karla mentioned one other thing that helped, and it may be something for both childbearing women and their doctors to keep in mind. She had to be asleep for her delivery, but an open-minded anesthesiologist allowed her husband—a nurse himself—to be in the operating room. "He was there the entire delivery," she told us, "and I felt like, 'Wow, God, this was your plan, because even though this is going on with my brain, you allowed him to be there.'" Like Jill, Karla was frustrated that she didn't get to see the birth for herself, but appreciated that the person she loved did—that he could have that moment of excitement and awe and pass it along to her when she woke up.

Finally, even for the vast majority of women, who will be awake—you might just feel a little loopy or dazed during birth—the pain of labor or the twists and turns of the day may understandably have unsettled you; an anesthetic or certain type of nausea medicine may have unseated temporarily your presence of mind. What I'd advise is that you make sure you get some space after delivery, carve out an opportunity for yourself and perhaps your partner too to reflect and gather what you remember as precious before it settles solidly into the past.

Remember that birth doesn't boil down to a moment in time, that birth stretches (in both directions) beyond the moment our children exit our bodies, that there are a multitude of moments that make up birth, moments for which we can and will want to be present. My good friend Jackie told me that what made the difference to her in her first birth—an unplanned cesarean in which she wasn't quite, in her words, "with it"—was waiting until she was more lucid to introduce her baby to the grandparents for the first time. She was the person to place her daughter Quinn into her father's outstretched arms. It was a moment in birth she will always remember—the stuff of birthing well, as far as both of us are concerned.

These moments emerge not just for women who were fuzzy or missed their deliveries either. My sister-in-law Diane (who was lucid for all four of her vaginal births) recalled with great affection what was among her favorite moments of all. She and my brother returned home from the hospital with their fourth—brand-new, their first boy. When they pulled up the driveway, my nieces—clad in princess costumes—poured out of the house to meet their new sibling, exclaiming, "Brother! Brother!" That, she told me, was something she wouldn't have missed for the world.

three

Personal Security

Ambiguous things can seem very threatening.

—MARY DOUGLAS

During idylls of safety, when your brain knows you are with someone you can trust, it needn't waste precious resources coping with stressors or menace. Instead it may spend its lifeblood learning new things or fine-tuning the process of healing. Its doors of perception swing wide open.

—DIANE ACKERMAN

Pamela is what we in obstetrics call a "grand multipara"—one of the few medical terms that connotes some sense of the magnificence of what has come before for the patient, the person—the birth of no fewer than six children.

I met Pam before she had any babies. She had thick brown hair, olive skin, dark eyes; to look at us, we could have been sisters, except for the fact that she towered over me by more than a foot. While I was her obstetrician, she gave birth to her first three gorgeously chubby baby boys. All were vaginal births, and breathtakingly quick. With her second, Seamus, she pushed just a few times before delivering him into my hastily gloved hands hovering over a freshly made hospital bed. Caleb, Pam's third, demanded similar haste, though his birth was most memorable for a moment when the world stopped, when his shoulder looked like it might be getting stuck behind Pam's pelvic bone. But the moment passed, the shoulder slipped out, and I handed Pam—who was even-keeled through it all—what turned out to be a strapping ten-pound boy.

What I learned from Pam, though, happened well after those births, after Caleb was out of diapers, after she had moved from North Carolina to Minnesota, was pregnant again, and had called me with a request for help, guidance, or maybe just an ear. Her obstetrician there was worried about the size of her babies, the possibility that the next one might be bigger and even more likely than Caleb to get stuck—and had suggested she consider a preemptive cesarean. "I'd do anything, of course, to keep my baby safe," she said, "but surgery, when labor takes all of fifteen minutes?" She reminded me that James, her first, was born not with a push, but a belly laugh from her that caused him to crown. Preemptive surgery just didn't make sense to her. It didn't make sense to me either.

But I knew what was going on. Her obstetrician was worried about something we all dread: shoulder dystocia. Not the momentary (if anxiety-provoking) pause that characterized Caleb's birth, but the terror of real dystocia, of the experience and sometimes the aftermath of a baby's being stuck, with its head delivered and body held up in its mother's body, its shoulder wedged behind an unmoving maternal bone. It is a harrowing obstetrical emergency, fortunately rare, and when it happens, the worst it usually entails is a traumatic memory, though it can lead to serious and permanent injury for childbearing women and their babies, even neonatal death. I'd been at my share of deliveries complicated by shoulder dystocia and understood the impulse, on her Minnesota obstetrician's part, to avoid it.

The problem is, we are pretty lousy at predicting when a dystocia will happen. There are some things that make it more likely—among them, a big baby, an overweight mom, the presence of diabetes, and of relevance to Pam, a history of more than one large infant. But a significant proportion of cases of dystocia happen with smaller babies who haven't a "risk factor" in sight. The worst dystocia I ever witnessed involved a petite first-time mom delivering a seven-pound baby girl. What this means is that the only way to completely avoid shoulder dystocia would be to do a cesarean on everyone. One study showed that even if everyone with a baby north of nine pounds had a cesarean, seventy-six cesareans would have to be done to avoid five cases of shoulder dystocia. Complicating matters is the fact that predicting the weight of babies near term is tricky, and a well-trained sonographer can be off by a pound or more in either direction. These handicaps aside, you'd still likely have to do thousands of otherwise unnecessary cesareans to prevent a single permanent injury related to shoulder dystocia, which nobody making policy thinks is a good idea.

The American College of Obstetricians and Gynecologists considered the data and concluded that a policy of preemptive cesareans isn't appropriate, though they conceded that planned cesarean delivery to prevent shoulder dystocia "may be considered" if a fetus is suspected of weighing eleven pounds or more in moms without diabetes (or ten pounds in women with diabetes). Pam wasn't close enough to her delivery date to determine whether this baby was going have a pound on ten-pound Caleb, but she told me she doubted it. This one, in fact, had felt smaller to her all along. And according to a couple of well-done studies (including one published in *The New England Journal of Medicine*), when it comes to estimating their fetus's weight, moms who have had one baby or more are at least as good as, and probably better than, doctors laying their hands on or—get this—trained sonographers with fancy machines.

No wonder Pam felt confused. I offered to talk with her doctor, who, as I suspected, had shoulder dystocia on his mind. He mentioned the events of Caleb's birth, which I assured him didn't get close to what we'd call a dystocia. And there was much to be reassured about—Pam was tall and her husband Jim was not (a discrepancy that has been shown to bode well for uncomplicated deliveries), she was thin, healthy, and—as obstetricians have been known to say to one another—you could drive a truck through her pelvis. (Not quite, but it was generous.) And besides, I told Pam's obstetrician, he probably wouldn't be able to justify an elective cesarean according to the profession's standards.

He conceded, and Pam told me later that they had agreed to go ahead with a trial of labor, but if anything seemed off track, the threshold for surgery would be low. I feared I knew what that meant too. All of a sudden, the power differential that has been written about time and again by critics of my profession came into sharp relief. I saw it, I felt it, I understood it: from my new vantage point, miles away from Pam's birth in Minnesota, it was crystal clear. Anything—a worrisome pattern on the fetal monitor, the appearance of "slow progress"—could mean she was headed down the hallway for the operating room. Her doctor would make the call and she wouldn't be in a position to press back, at least not hard enough to matter. Someone might, but not Pam. Her primary concern was for everyone to be safe, and questioning her physician's mid-labor judgment call about the health of her baby or the likelihood of dystocia wasn't something that would make her feel safer in the least.

What Pam's experience did for me was shift the presumption that access to technology necessarily meant that patients were safer when it came to childbirth. In all likelihood, Pam was going to end up with a cesarean (that she didn't need)—not because her doctor wanted money or was impatient or even was afraid of lawsuits, but because his aversion to risk for a patient he cared about centered on the unlikely but real possibility of a particular obstetrical emergency that he could handily avoid with an operation he was really good at doing. This woman, I thought—empirically speaking—isn't any safer in the hospital than she would be at home. In fact, access to technology was *the* pressing threat. And given that she wanted to keep having babies (and that cesarean adds risks to future pregnancies and births), the risk a preemptive surgery would entail would last a reproductive lifetime.

Up to this point, I had thought about out-of-hospital birth as akin to riding a bike (indeed, a motorcycle) without a helmet—that women's decisions to eschew mainstream obstetrical care were about an unfathomable weighting of experience over safety. Indeed, I had been flummoxed by the notion that the women who chose out-of-hospital birth thought something was more important than safeguarding their own health or that of their children (and I was curious, to boot, to know what that something was).

But while such is the story often understood by my colleagues in obstetrics, whose interface with out-of-hospital births is most often with those that have gone badly, there is another way to understand women's choices about birth location. It's not about trading off safety for some abstract notion of a "good" or meaningful birth; it's not a question of selfishness versus responsibility. It's all *about* safety—about feeling safe in the context of profound physically and existentially vulnerable moments of their life. Thus, perhaps it is no surprise that one of the most prevalent considerations raised by women across the Good Birth Project—whatever their birth location—was how important safety is to having a good birth. But assurance of physical well-being, central as it is to a good birth, is just a part of what wise women say a safe birth means. As you'll see, this turned out to be the case for Pam. But before we get to the end of her story, let's consider how safety has manifested for the women of the Good Birth Project.

Understanding Safety

When we listen to women, we hear how important safety is. But their stories suggest a broader and richer conception of safety than is often understood or discussed. For one thing, they reflect differences (between one woman and another, between women and doctors) in understandings of which risks loom largest and matter most. Women's voices sharpen our focus on what is centrally at stake in finding our way to a good birth—not agreement on some empirical threshold of acceptable risk, not the impossible elimination of the unthinkable, but instead a need to feel safe and, perhaps more to the point, *secure* in the context of birth, despite the uncertainties it inevitably entails. And it turns out that aspirations toward such personal security are not unique to patients, but shape in important ways the language and actions of all who interface with, advocate for, and argue about what it is that makes for a good birth. They lead clear-eyed and honest professionals on either side of the birth wars to disagree about what makes for a responsible birth, to come to different conclusions about the same study and how it relates to patients, to advocate for divergent guidelines and approaches to birth—and to insist and believe with whole hearts that it is they who have women's and children's health in mind.

What I mean by *personal security* is what ethicists Ruth Faden and Madison Powers described in their 2006 book, *Social Justice*: "human interests everyone has in maintaining physical and bodily integrity and psychological inviolability." Birth, of course, brings these interests to a head, challenges our grip on them, and ultimately demands that we reformulate our ideas about them. When we listen to women reflecting on their births, we hear five ways that women navigate personal security. Physical safety is the first and arguably most prominent component of personal security, but there are two other pieces to it. One is the trio of things I think of together: comfort, privacy, and calmness. And the other is trust.

As I talk about what these things mean to women, it will become clear that they are not entirely separable, but rather overlapping and intertwined. You will also see echoes of *agency*, and previews of other concepts we'll address later in the book. Further, the distinction between the physical and psychological is somewhat artificial. *Feeling* or *believing* that you are physically safe is of course a psychological state, not a fact of the matter. And the feeling that we are inviolable, psychologically speaking, will require a measure of safety in the physical sense of the word. But I will take as my starting point how women parse notions of security; what comes forth in their stories, I hope, will be a source of wisdom for you. I'll begin with what they say about the thorny question of physical safety.

Physical Safety

I think that it's absolutely important for the person who's having the baby to try and have the baby in a place they feel is safe. And if that's a hospital, for a lot of people that is the best place, because they feel safe in a hospital. But there are other options.

—Maya

It almost goes without saying that a good birth is, at the very least, a safe birth, and so I devote much of this chapter to the notion of safety in the traditional sense of the word—as distance, or freedom, from risk of bodily harm.

Defined as such, safety might seem at first glance to be something concrete and objective—raising the question of what women who have been through birth could possibly tell us about its meaning. Shouldn't well-done research studies of birth outcomes tell us what a safe birth is? The answer, in short, is no.

The first reason is that the professions differ—and differ widely—on what lessons should be drawn from research on all manner of questions pertaining to birth. Take for instance debate about birth location. The medical community's long-standing opposition to home birth is based on its assessment that dreaded if rare outcomes are less frequent when women give birth in a hospital. The midwifery and public health communities dispute these data and point to strong evidence that medical interventions themselves impose significant morbidities on what is a physiologically normal event. Short of simply taking sides, which I don't think is wise, women approaching birth need to figure out what safety means to them amid these often opposing views—something we'll get into much more, later in this chapter and the book.

The second reason is that studies alone can't point a clear line to a safe birth. Even where professions agree, women themselves have choices to make and options here will involve weighing probabilities of things that may or may not happen and that strike different women differently. For instance, many women who have given birth by cesarean will have two options before them in a subsequent pregnancy: they can have another cesarean or they can attempt vaginal birth. There is some consensus—even between midwives and doctors—that both options are reasonable in many circumstances. For women who dread the unlikely but real possibility of *emergency* cesarean, a planned cesarean might feel safest. For other women, keeping the greatest distance from any cesarean—elective or emergent—might feel like the safe route, so planning a VBAC (vaginal birth after cesarean) may strike them as the safest choice. Understanding what we value and how we feel about risk and uncertainty will be critical to finding safety in birth.

And the third reason is that being safe and feeling safe are different things. The sort of safety I'm talking about here is not an objective measure—it is decidedly subjective; it is linked to a woman's sense that what strikes her as dreadful is at the greatest distance possible. It is often inversely related to fear. A good outcome doesn't mean that a birth was safe, nor does it mean that it *felt* safe. Women told us how brushes with danger—even those in which actual physical harm was negligible—remain front and center as they think back on their births. As I emphasized in Chapter 1, a good outcome and a good birth, while often concomitant, are not one and the same. Rather, *feeling* safe in birth—comfortably distant from risk—is one of the things that women describe as crucial to a good birth.

Women are not alone in their need to feel safe. What all we professionals (doctors and midwives alike) really want to do is eliminate risk—to snub out risk in birth. And so we doctors try to manage it by naming it, zeroing in on it, monitoring everything we can, and deploying our tools to try to contain it. Midwives emphasize that birth itself is "normal, natural, and safe" and that we should trust the pregnant body, that it was "meant" to birth and birth well. But we can never be totally free of risk—in birth no less than in life generally. Overfocusing on deleting the last increments of risk, as doctors may tend to do, or overemphasizing trust of the pregnant body, as midwives may tend to do, may mean overlooking the inescapability of risk, and together these approaches leave childbearing women with a stark choice between two ways of thinking about safety in birth that hardly account for what they themselves experience and understand.

It turns out that women's views of safety in birth are considerably more nuanced than either profession's received view. For many of the women of the Good Birth Project, safety in birth was found not in absolute assurances, but in their ability to buttress a sense of personal security up against the things that emerge as most threatening. This means that the definition of safety requires not just understanding what risks are "out there" but looking in and grasping what it is that moves you, what things strike you as threatening or comforting, what would make you feel safe in birth.

To see what I mean, let's turn back to the hotly debated topic of out-of-hospital birth and a handful of wise women's reflections on their choices of birth location. Two women we've heard from already, Liz and Raquel, shared a particular definition of safety, but it was very different from the way that two others, Vicky and Maisie, thought about it. Each woman's notion of safety shaped her choice about where to give birth and her reflections on those choices later. For mother of two Liz (introduced in Chapter 1), feelings of safety derived from the structured environment of the hospital, choice of delivery date, and close monitoring of her and her baby. She notes:

> I felt very safe the first time around, because, actually, I think
> with it being induced . . . it was so structured and I felt like it was
> so monitored, you know; the baby's heartbeat was monitored
> and I was monitored and there were people coming in to check
> on a regular basis.

Raquel, introduced in Chapter 2, had a similar definition of safety. After three vaginal births—all of which required a big tug with forceps after hours of pushing—she chose to deliver by cesarean for her last to avoid the long-term consequences that a fourth vaginal tear might entail.

> I have always felt like I wanted all these interventions. I read on websites, women don't want an IV, and I'm thinking, "I want an IV." They don't want internal fetal monitoring—they see that as a negative. I think, "You better believe I want my baby monitored." I want the baby monitored; I want myself monitored. I had different complications—I want those managed well. You know, the idea of giving birth at home would be totally negative to me . . . Who says, "My C-section was my best birth?" But that's me.

Interestingly enough, the very things that made Liz and Raquel feel safe were viewed as threatening by Vicky, who gave birth four times in a free-standing birth center:

> I think I always felt very safe at the birthing center. I always felt like I was in a place . . . where nobody was going to try and force anything on me I didn't want. Sometimes when you read about birth preparation, it sounds like you're preparing for battle—you're preparing to resist all interventions. And that was why I wanted to be at the birthing center, because I didn't want to have to do battle when I was in labor, and so I always felt like the midwives and I were very much on the same page. And I always felt very safe.

We hear echoes of *agency* in Vicky's statement, but what's particularly important here is that the prospect of losing that agency made her feel unsafe. Maisie (also introduced in Chapter 1), whose third birth was at home, shared Vicky's concern about the threat of intervention, which loomed so large that the hospital seemed like a space full of danger. She put it this way:

> In a hospital, you're always wondering, "Okay, am I progressing fast enough? Are things going the way they want it to? Is that

little readout in that machine doing everything right? Did I turn the wrong way? Is it picking up something that's not right? Is everything going as planned?" Because all I'm thinking is "They're going to want to cut me open. They're going to want to take a knife to me." Whether it's an episiotomy or a cesarean or whatever, they're too quick with the knife, and that scares me. That's not safe to me.

All of these women's views make sense. The risks that people reasonably notice, the risks that move them, will vary from person to person.

For some women, safety will mean minimizing the (already low) risks of very bad things—risks, admittedly, that loom large for me. As a doctor, I've been too close to too many of these sorts of risks—a handful of obstetrical emergencies over the past two decades that, but for immediate access to medicine's resources, would have ended in loss of life, or a harrowing brush with it. I've had my socks soaked by the blood of a mother whose hemorrhage after birth was compared by those who witnessed it to the flow of water from a hydrant. I've looked at the gray faces of colleagues who had resuscitated a formerly healthy mom who labored for just an hour, then stopped breathing moments after giving birth due to a blood clot that a last push had dislodged from her pelvis and sent to her lungs. Such moments, practically unthinkable and fortunately rare, are definitive for some women for whom a good birth is premised on a feeling of safety or security from ready access to technology and lifesaving equipment.

This does not mean that hospitals always feel safe to me—not in the least. Rather, it means that while I take seriously the threats within their walls, those threats seem more manageable than those I'd face outside. Such was the lesson of the birth of my third son, Charlie, back in 2004.

I remember a lightning-bolt moment of terror in that delivery, in the midst of my cesarean. I had grown an enormous baby, estimated at over ten pounds, surrounded by more than the usual share of amniotic fluid (I had been accused by a mother of triplets of being one of her select crowd). Weeks in advance, I'd made all the arrangements: a repeat cesarean scheduled on a numerically notable birth date, with my favorite nurse, nurse anesthetist, and obstetrician in attendance. I was overtaken by contractions, of course, a full twenty-four hours before the scheduled time.

In the operating room, my colleagues took their time opening my abdomen and uterus. Initially during the procedure, with Kim at my side, I had some success blocking out the conversation over the blue drape—unsettling as fingernails on a chalkboard—about the inside of my open belly, interspersed with the equally hair-raising high-pitched buzz of the Bovie cautery—an electrical knife of sorts used in surgery that buzzes (and stops bleeding) as it cuts. I also somehow managed to avoid engaging with the swell of voices that accompanied the breaking of my amniotic sac and subsequent tidal wave of fluid that I imagined spouted like a geyser through the hole they made in my overdistended uterus, across the drape, onto the surgeon's boots, and then the floor. But then Laura, the utterly competent, reassuringly conservative surgeon, asked for a vacuum.

I knew too much to ignore that the request meant trouble. And to this day, I do not know whether I was literally screaming or silent as I was overtaken by terror—terror that there was a moment in which my obstetrician wasn't sure she could get my baby out with her hands. He was enormous, his head was floating out of my pelvis, and she needed something to get it through the hole she had sliced in my uterus. For a moment, however fleeting, I encountered the terror of losing my baby—losing him before I'd met him, before I'd become his mother. The moment passed, and the order of the world seemed to come back into place, especially once they pressed Charlie's cheek against my own. But in some ways that moment will never really be over, not in my lifetime anyway, not for me. In familiar surroundings, with all the tools of my trade in the competent hands of colleagues, I did not feel safe—that birth entailed way too close a brush with bodily harm to my new boy.

Whatever could the lesson be? What would make me feel safe?

One possible answer would be to steer clear of the operating room. But if I was ever to have a baby again (and I planned to), that wouldn't be possible. Given the comfort I continued to reap from ready access to lifesaving technology, walking away from the hospital into the arms of a midwife wouldn't help matters. Neither would trying to give birth vaginally, even in a hospital, since I also find comfort in evidence, and there is almost none about what happens when women like me with three prior cesareans attempt a VBAC. In short, a fourth cesarean was the only sort of birth that I could conceive of as safe; but now, after the moment of terror I'd experienced when Laura asked for the vacuum, a fourth cesarean felt scary.

In the years that followed, the answer became clear. To this day, that utterly competent surgeon—who was not for a moment afraid during my cesarean—talks about what a small incision she was able to make; there is no mention of the fact that it made more difficult the task of pulling out my child. But what I live with is a different scar. The small incision that Laura viewed with pride meant something else to me—it was in its diminutive length a reminder of a moment I wish I could forget, that gave me considerable pause about my next delivery. I could have talked to Laura about it, tried to get her to understand my view. Instead, for William's birth I concluded that what would make me feel safe was to find someone else. I told my new doctor about that moment in Charlie's birth, how it had stayed with me, how important it was to me that she not struggle in getting my baby out, how delighted I'd be with a wide incision and an easy delivery.

Echoes of my experience ran throughout the Good Birth interviews. Like me, Raquel was attuned to the risks that technology could address, but for different reasons. For her the threat of things going wrong was not an idle one. Her own experiences were evidence enough that pregnant bodies are not predictably healthy and normal—that pregnancy is not to be trusted. For one, each time she reached thirty-six weeks she developed preeclampsia, a physiologically mysterious and not uncommon condition that complicates about 6 to 8 percent of pregnancies. It is marked by high blood pressure and protein in the urine and, if untreated, can lead in rare cases to seizures and even death. Most of the time it is easily treated with an infusion of magnesium through an IV, and cured by delivery (as it was each time for Raquel). But what most derailed Raquel's trust in the pregnant body were a series of miscarriages. Each imparted a profound sense of loss, "the feeling," as she put it, "that your body has failed you." Medicine's tools at the ready gave her the feeling that she could get through birth safely—they made her feel secure.

Other women notice more likely risks—the risks the midwifery community has argued a hospital birth can entail. For Vicky, the pressing threat was *unwanted* intervention—the IV or epidural she felt she'd have to resist if she were in a conventional hospital setting. For Maisie, the pressing threat was *unnecessary* intervention—the cesarean or episiotomy that she could do without, and would do without if she kept her distance from a physician. Given a cesarean rate topping 30 percent in the United States, Maisie's concern is far from unfounded. Most of us agree that some portion of cesareans done these days aren't completely justified (we differ on how many and which ones), and public health efforts are under way to reduce their overall rate, while consumer advocates press hospitals to be more transparent about their cesarean statistics. Finally, there is the threat of medical error that is arguably more likely when birth happens in a hospital. The Institute of Medicine estimated that up to 98,000 deaths per year in the United States—in medical patients in general, that is—can be attributed to medical error. It's what captured mother of three Carmen's attention (she gave birth at home, in a birthing center, and in the hospital): "At the hospital, I felt plenty safe in terms of an emergency happening. I was just afraid that [laughs] an emergency would be created." Distance from these risks—in a home or freestanding birth center—helped make each of these women feel safe, secure, and remote from the things that emerged for them as most threatening.

There are others who have one notion of safety, but have to readjust—like the women Stella sees. Stella is a maternal-fetal medicine specialist who routinely cares for women with bleeding disorders, heart problems, and sometimes double-digit chances of death in the context of birth. Once a midwife herself, she talked about how seeing her high-risk patients through these harrowing circumstances changed her own criteria for a good birth.

> For me as a provider for very high risk patients, [a good birth] is when—given a set of circumstances that the possibility, or perhaps even the probability, was that things were not going to be good, that the natural history of the condition, for either the mother or the baby, was that one's life or health would be jeopardized—the good birth is when we can change the natural history of a bad outcome and make it good. Or we can get the best outcome in bad circumstances.
>
> So, for me it's different than it was when I was a midwife, where a good birth was the spontaneous vaginal delivery of the

term baby, with the unmedicated mother, with the intact perineum, with the placenta that didn't have to be removed, and the recovery that didn't involve an infection or a hemorrhage. I mean, that was the kind of a perfect birth. And so now that that isn't the bulk of my practice, my criteria are different. So for me it's the premature baby where we got the steroids in place, but the baby goes to the intensive care nursery and doesn't have to be intubated and doesn't have a head bleed. And I see the baby five years later and the baby is perfectly on target developmentally and . . . and that's a thrill.

For Stella, safety's moving goalposts emerge most vividly when she compares her past experience as a midwife with her current perspective as a high-risk obstetrician. But the shift can come up in the midst of birth too. It did for my friend Joanie, who started labor in a birth center but transferred to the hospital after a couple of hours, when she started bleeding. She ultimately underwent cesarean—and as she tells it, her midwife's insistence that she get moved to the front of the long line of women awaiting surgery that night is what saved her and her now twelve-year-old's life. "At that moment," she told me, "I wouldn't have cared if they told me they had to deliver Hayden out of my nose." You might be surprised to hear, though, that Joanie gave birth to her next two children back in the birth center, with no complications. The goalposts had shifted back.

Ultimately, the lesson is that safety won't be found in simply pressing risk away, imagining it doesn't exist, or in blindly relying on technology to keep us safe in birth. Rather, it requires looking inside, understanding which risks matter most, and envisioning how they might best be managed. When it comes to safety in birth, it is not that anything goes. But a woman's sense of safety—the distance she perceives between herself and harm—depends on what's come before, what strikes her as most threatening, what her circumstances are. Safety can't be traced to a particular birthplace or mode or even series of events, expected or not. What safety means for Stella's "high-risk" patients will be different from what it means for women she took care of when she was a midwife. For many of us, though, pregnancy is neither immediately life-threatening, nor is it eminently safe.

I can't tell you what a safe birth is, and neither can any of the wise women who shared their experiences. What I can say is that safety is something that requires looking inside, understanding what risks move you, and how best to keep them at bay.

Safety will mean one thing to me as a doctor. It will look different to someone who has had bad experiences in a hospital in a prior birth—or even in an event unrelated to birth: a family member who has had a surgical complication, a friend who has had a child die, a colleague who has suffered from overuse of technology.

Safety will also shift according to how you think about risk. My friend Jackie blames her father—a malpractice attorney—for cultivating her aversion to risk. "If I knew the chances of my having problems with delivery were infinitesimal," she told me, "I'd still go to the hospital, because I figure it'd just be my luck to fall into that tiny category." Experience can have a similar effect. In her gorgeous memoir on pregnancy loss, *An Exact Replica of a Figment of My Imagination*, Elizabeth McCracken puts it this way: "Once you've been on the losing side of great odds, you never find statistics comforting again." Women with a history of reproductive loss or infertility may feel not only that they can't trust birth's normalcy, but that risk, in their life, will not pay attention to the odds. Perhaps some would call this irrational, but women's relationship with risk will shape the way they experience birth—as dangerous or safe. And in the end, women tell us, that feeling of safety is crucial.

Comfort, Privacy, and Calmness

What are the things that make you comfortable if you're in pain? Because labor is pain. Labor is work. Otherwise it would be called picnic. What are the things that make you feel more comfortable? A lavender candle, certain music, a rice sock to your back, holding your teddy bear, a certain blanket? You know, what are those things that make you feel comfortable? And even though you might be hurting, what are the things that are going to make you feel at ease, that you can do that work?

—DONNA, MIDWIFE

Now suppose you've made peace with the idea of risk in birth—or, at least you've identified the place and approach in which the risks that matter to you feel as comfortably distant as imaginable. Personal security in birth, for most people, requires more. For most women, it requires the right combination of comfort, privacy, and calmness that together help us feel at ease. If unsurprising at first blush, some women find these things to be surprisingly out of reach in birth, or within reach in places and situations they'd never imagined.

Take thirty-eight-year-old Kyra, a first-time mom whom we interviewed before and after she gave birth. Kyra's primary concern aside from a healthy delivery was to be in what felt to her like a comfortable, private, calm environment. She decided to give birth in her home, with her husband, her midwife, and her twin sister by her side. Yet over the course of her labor, her comfort in that space started to unravel.

Kyra had always been the caregiver, nurturing her sister, her husband, and their dogs. In birth, she found she needed someone to care for her. Yet her husband and sister, taking seriously their new roles, began arguing over what was best for Kyra: when and how to blow up the inflatable tub, which tea to brew, how much to worry when the person they loved seemed to be getting exhausted and withdrawn.

We'd interviewed Kyra before her birth, and presciently she'd noted that the one thing that would make her birth a bad experience would be if "there was a lot of tension, a lot of strife, if there were arguing or . . . anger coming into it. I think all of those things would taint it for me." Home for her had always been a place of tranquillity and peace, but her being in a space of need disrupted that dynamic in a way none of her family members anticipated.

When complications developed, she ultimately went to the hospital by helicopter, where she was surprised to find great comfort and relief—notably in the moments before her sister and husband (who had to get themselves to the hospital in a car on winding roads) arrived to join her in the hospital room. Part of that came from physical comfort she found in a well-made hospital bed (compared with the hard board on which she'd been transported): "I just remember how soft the bed felt—it felt like I was being suspended in the coziest, comfiest [laughs]—after being on that board." But part of it was the comfort of a new space in which she could feel at ease.

At that point, just being by myself, in that room, and [the nurse] was there, quietly moving around—that was like the absolute easiest time of the whole birth . . . That's what made me think maybe what happened with just [my sister's and husband's] emotions and their feelings and everything around it, seeing me in that state, really affected it. I just remember things being easy in that room. It wasn't even hard to go through the contractions. So that was kind of interesting.

So what can we learn from Kyra's experience? At first glance, the wisdom she reaped seems specific to her: that as much as she loves home, in giving birth she required something else, and she found it in a hospital. Yet others *will* find a sense of security at home, or in a birthing center. The question of course is why—and, can we figure it out before we get there? I'd offer that we can—but it will take some work to understand what that secure feeling requires—what comfort, privacy and calmness mean and what they do for us in birth.

Comfort

There is nothing comfortable, really, about giving birth, however you do it. We have long dispensed with the notion that contractions are appropriately described as "rushes" (as they once were by famous midwife Ina May Gaskin and others who thought it useful to de-emphasize that labor hurts). And what we do in birth involves such intimacy, such potential exposure, that other meanings of "comfortable"—like being at ease—would seem at first blush just as ill-suited to birth as the terms once used to cloak its often racking sensations.

And yet one of the things women most frequently said they needed or wanted in birth was comfort—in at least two senses of the word. Some talk about physical comfort and focus on freedom from or adequate management of pain. For others, comfort is more like an emotional state—feeling consoled, reassured, given solace or relief.

Mother of four Eloise, forty-three, used the term *comfort* simply to describe freedom from pain. When we asked her what she thought was most important to a good birth, she answered, "Being comfortable," and went on to reflect that the pain she endured before her epidural kicked in was among the bad moments in her good birth.

To the extent that *comfort* is a word Eloise used, as we do often in medicine, to describe simply the absence of pain, it doesn't say much about security. But to the extent that being in physical pain is experienced by some of us—especially in birth—as threatening to bodily or psychological integrity, the link between comfort and personal security is clear. And it turns out that many women made that connection in reflecting how important comfort was to their having a good birth.

Recall Natalie, from Chapter 2, who had given birth once without anesthesia and was, over the course of her second pregnancy, trying to figure out whether to do the same this time around. Natalie had wanted—needed—the tussle with pain in her first birth. In that birth, pain had meaning for her; fighting it was her way of showing that the "doctors were wrong." But in her second birth, she ultimately got an epidural and loved the way it allowed her to relax.

> The anesthesiologist came in and she did the epidural, and they broke the waters, and then it was just so great. I was so happy. I was sitting back there after all of that initial chaos and after I got comfortable and, "God," I told my husband, "this is so great." And I was so happy. And I was relaxed. And I know that helped me to progress. I really do. I can look back and say the reason my first labor probably took so long is I wasn't relaxed.

Secure in her physical comfort (and perhaps in the notion that she didn't need to prove that she could win that tussle with pain), she was able to "enjoy" her birth and attend to it more completely.

For others, comfort meant not the absence of pain but its adequate management, often linked with their ability to cope with it. Such was the case with May, who gave birth with a midwifery group in a hospital setting and spoke of "comfort measures."

> My midwife that day was awesome . . . She helped me do things that my doula hadn't helped me do last time, with dancing,

working with my hips, different types of comfort techniques and measures I had never even seen before that really helped me cope.

If coping is the effort to manage something taxing, we see again the natural link to personal security. Comfort, then, emerges as a way to keep oneself together in the context of physically painful labor. Pain that is managed, and manageable, can make us feel not only comfortable but also personally secure.

Kyra was after something different when she talked about comfort, but that notion was no less tied to personal security. She knew that giving birth at home would involve a certain amount of physical discomfort; what she wanted was to be in an environment where she could "relax the most . . . where we can do the things that are most comfortable for us so we are in the best place emotionally and physically to birth this child." Comfort was about being at ease emotionally.

But walls—even those that are familiar and strong—do not necessarily a safe space make. What we also need is to ask whether the space we choose will give us comfort *in birth*.

When my husband and I first got married, we both were working pretty long hours, being doctors. When both of us were home, it felt like a wonderful relief to me; we were finally in a place where we could relax, together— except when Kim was on call. Since I was still in residency, *on call* for me meant long nights in the hospital, and I wasn't allowed off the premises. Kim, on the other hand, was junior faculty and could take calls from home, which I perceived as a luxury. Over time, though, I realized it wasn't. When that beeper was on his belt, he'd be home, but his tie was on, and he sat on the edge of his seat; his back rarely graced the pillows that lined our oversize chair. Home didn't feel comfortable to him at all. It turned out, when he was on call, it was much more fun to be with him in the hospital, where he felt at ease. Despite its comforts (generous chairs, chocolate chip cookies), home wasn't a comfortable space for him (or me) when he wore his doctor's hat.

It's a helpful, if imperfect, analogy. It's not about whether you feel comfortable at home, but whether you can find comfort there when you are giving birth. Sometimes comfort will come from a beloved space or a familiar pillow. Sometimes comfort can be found in other objects that reassure.

For instance, in each of the rooms at our local birth center is a beautiful rocking chair. Each looks hand-carved, and they all have wide seats and worn armrests that betray the hundreds of women's hands that have gripped them while giving birth, the hundreds of elbows that have rested with a new babe in arms. For some, these chairs will signal comfort in their shape—or in the reminder that so many others have labored well there before. For others, these chairs, if gorgeous artifacts, will appear hard and unfamiliar, or *too* worn. Whether they appear to be a source of comfort or alienation will depend on what they evoke for the woman anticipating birth.

But as Kyra discovered when her husband and sister began to argue, comfort also derives from our interactions with the people around us. In birth, we want to be known, feel loved, feel *cared for*; that, of course, makes us feel secure. I'll get into this more in Chapter 4, when I talk about connectedness, but it's important to understand that there is a link between comfort and how we relate to others in the moment. Such was the case for Malia, who gave birth in a community hospital for her first birth and a birth center the second time around. Comfort came from the sense that she was known, that she was among friends, that she would not be abandoned in birth, endowing a sense of personal security. What made her birth-center birth good, she said, was a sense of security that came from "having somebody attend to my birth who I felt like I had a relationship with, who I knew. I mean, it felt like going in there with a bunch of old friends, so it made it a much more comfortable experience."

Still others used the term *comfort* to connote the feeling that came from being reassured by people they felt were competent, knowledgeable, or committed to their well-being. Mother of two Lindsey noted that her midwife was "so attentive at the birth and making sure I was okay and the baby was okay [that] my comfort level just rose . . . I think that is what made it a good experience for me."

We see the need for comfort come up against birth's challenges to our security: our bodies will necessarily be breached; we need physical comfort; our identities will be transformed and integrity challenged; we need consolation and reassurance in the midst of transition. For some, comfort will be found in the pharmacologic relief of pain or a personal triumph over it. For others, it will be found in a familiar space, in caring practitioners, in reminders of who we are and hope to be.

Privacy

In addition to comfort, time and again women also talked about the importance of privacy—their need to be free from unwanted intrusions. Birth can be among the most intimate of life events, and the entry of unwelcome visitors will feel to many like a threat to their security—even a violation.

This is the word Sally tried to resist using when she described her first birth, during which the use of forceps in an academic medical center drew what felt like an oppressive and intrusive crowd.

> With my son, I remember being . . . [sigh] I don't know what the word is. I wouldn't say "violated," because really at that point I just didn't care. But I can remember opening my eyes and at one point I can tell you there had to have been fourteen people in the room, because apparently they don't do forceps very often, so it's this big thing. "Hey, forceps. Go get the janitor. Let's everybody look." I just remember opening my eyes and seeing all these people and then shutting them again, going, "I cannot focus on that." So part of my plan [for my second] was that I didn't want—I forget how I phrased it—but basically we didn't want a circus.

When Carol planned her first birth at home, privacy was key to her reasoning. The privacy that home would afford, she thought, would allow her to feel secure enough to let herself go and not worry what other people might be thinking.

> It's definitely me being in a very different position than I've ever been in before, so having an environment where I feel able to do that [is important]. In the hospital, the rooms aren't soundproof— there are going to be other people that are going to be hearing whatever I'm doing, and I don't want to be self-conscious. I think

that will affect how much I can relax and allow my body to do what it's going to do.

Like Carol, Maisie appreciated in retrospect that, being in the privacy of her own home, she could be herself, unafraid of embarrassment, secure in her post-birth reverie.

So with [my fourth baby], I was just sitting there on a birth stool, holding her, nursing her, looking at her, sun shining through the blinds, blood all over the kitchen floor [laughs], and it didn't matter. It was just neat. And I wasn't embarrassed or uncomfortable or going, "Did I make a fool of myself in front of strangers?" And there was no insecurity.

For several other women, privacy meant freedom, not just from the intrusions of strangers, but from the immediate attention (and potentially the worry) of loved ones who might be genuinely supportive and interested. Mother of five Paula put it this way:

I'm not one who wants an audience while birthing. I just like to be left alone. So I wouldn't want a friend to take pictures and another friend to do this and another—no, I wasn't that way. Midwife, my husband—that's the end of it. That's how we had it. I'm not ashamed either. Some people have [their] kids there. I couldn't do that. No, I would be their mom. They shouldn't be put in a position like that where they think they have to protect me.

Finally, some women's need for privacy was about maintaining a space of intimacy with their partner. Such was the case for Alex, who gave birth three times in a freestanding birthing center.

I really enjoyed that time [leading up to the birth]. Because, like I said, it was private. The midwives were very good at allowing us to use that space . . . just having that quiet time leading up to the baby getting here, because that's your last little bit of quiet time.

The right amount of privacy in birth will be different for different women—it requires figuring out when someone's presence will feel helpful or celebratory, and when it might cross the line to intrusion. Birth exposes us—physically and emotionally. If you are looking toward birth, think about whom you want to share that with, and whether you can be yourself with the people you consider asking (or allowing) across the threshold. The presence of a relative stranger whose job it is to assist (like a doula or nurse) might help you maintain a sense of privacy better than a loved one who feels—to you— out of place. Finally, remember that, like comfort, birth requires a certain sort of privacy that—depending on whom you want around—can be found in the birthing center, hospital, or home.

Calmness

Women also talk about the importance of calmness and the ways in which chaos can cast an indelible pall, can eliminate their sense of personal security—even in births in which the ultimate outcome was good.

Such was the case for Mara. She had studied Lamaze, and her mom— who'd had a euphoric home birth in the early 1970s—had encouraged her to give "natural birth" a go. Nearly a week overdue, she found herself stuck between wanting to let nature take its course and let labor begin on its own, and wanting her husband, who had to return to a military base out of state, by her side. She chose the latter, and her doctor agreed to induce labor at forty-one weeks.

As is often the case with induced labor, a day's worth of contractions had not budged her cervix. Then, she told us, "All of a sudden, I felt wetness, down there. And I reached down and it was just all blood." Concerned about the likely possibility that the placenta had separated from the uterine wall (we call this an abruption, and it can lead to very heavy and dangerous bleeding), the doctor quickly decided to do a cesarean; and Mara's birth went from calm to terrifyingly chaotic.

> I was crying, Jake was crying, and it wasn't just about the C-section. It was because the baby seemed sick, his heart rate was just staying down, my [oxygen levels] were dropping, and it was just so scary. They thought I was abrupting—they thought

I was bleeding out . . . They didn't even tell my husband where we were going. They just threw everything onto the bed and ran to the operating room, and [my son] was out in under two min-utes . . . It was just sort of a chaotic moment and we kind of thought we wouldn't have another one after that, because it was so scary and sad.

Mara decided in her second birth that calmness was absolutely key. One might think she'd turn away from the hospital and find a midwife whom she trusted to coax her baby out in a dimly lit space. But for Mara, vaginal birth after cesarean entailed the real possibility of an emergent transition to surgi-cal birth; and that sort of chaos—fresh, almost palpable—was what she needed to avoid. So she decided on a repeat cesarean, a week ahead of her due date. Reflecting on her second birth, she noted:

There wasn't any scariness—we went in and in two hours we had a baby to enjoy, and we planned for everything, and it was just altogether different, in a better way, I think . . . I really enjoyed it. I mean honestly, I look forward to having another scheduled C-section, where I would never look forward to another labor process.

It is no wonder that women embrace a certain amount of calmness in birth. Liz, who without hesitation chose hospital birth, nevertheless appreci-ated how a calm atmosphere signaled that she was safe, not sick.

You don't really want to feel like you're sick. And so it was im-portant for me to feel like the atmosphere in the room was calm-ing, and we had music playing . . . So it was just a very soothing experience.

It is important to point out that, just because a birth might be complicated, it does not mean that it cannot be calm. Jill, introduced in Chapter 2—who had a rare and life-threatening complication of pregnancy known as "acute fatty liver"—also appreciated the calm atmosphere in the face of the unthinkable.

> Everybody was just very caring, and it just gave me calmness about it. Nobody was rushing around and screaming and panicking and they all seemed to know what they were doing, and I just felt that I was in good hands.

Calmness was celebrated, not just in its function as a buttress against the life-threatening, but as a good in itself. Natalie found this to be true of her second birth, in which she opted for an epidural.

> It was a really, really good experience, and not at all what I expected. It was very peaceful. It was very gentle, which it wasn't for my first. For [my first] I see the bright lights and all the doctors and I remember the pain. [For my second] I don't know if all the lights were off in the room, but in my mind the lights were off, and there was a serenity to it. And yeah, there were lights on, but it was—sounds really dumb—more like the glow of a fireplace. It had that kind of warmth about the room and I felt that kind of sense. The second experience was a lot more positive.

No doubt if you watch births on television or have heard about them from friends, it may seem like calmness is an elusive goal, and it can be. Still, it's worth thinking about how to clear the way for it. If you have a high-intensity doctor—or a high-intensity family member—consider how that might make you feel in labor and think about enlisting help to keep things calm.

By virtue of his surgical training, Kim has an abundance of what my historically minded medical colleagues would call *aequanimitas*. It is a term evoked by "father of modern medicine" and Johns Hopkins professor William Osler to describe a certain mode of doctoring or being, an "imperturbability" characterized by "coolness and presence of mind under all circumstances, calmness amid storm, clearness of judgment in moments of grave peril, immobility, impassiveness, or, to use an old and expressive word, *phlegm*." Some people want their husbands to cry when they give birth; let's just say I preferred phlegm to tears.

My friend Jackie is also a rock of sorts. Her sister Denise invited her to be a part of her recent birth, not just because she adored and appreciated Jackie's company, but also so that she would run interference with their malpractice-attorney dad and her overly anxious mother-in-law. Neither was allowed anywhere near Denise and her husband during labor—Denise had the prescience to know that either would pull apart the tenuous calm they'd crafted in anticipation of delivery.

Of course, you can shore up calm in other ways. Keeping things calm was part of Mara's decision to have a second cesarean; it was part of what Natalie found so satisfying about birth with an epidural. It is something others find in well-supported labor in birthing centers and homes, in tubs filled with water that lifts the belly and the spirit, in spaces where they feel safe and secure.

Trust

> *Without trust, what matters to me would be unsafe, unless like the Stoic I attach myself only to what can thrive, or be safe from harm, however others act.*
>
> —ANNETTE BAIER, PHILOSOPHER

> *It's that feeling of security that you're taken care of. Now it might be very scary and it might hurt and it might be unpredictable . . . but I think that's why you just want to look up at your doctor and your nurses and have that feeling like, "I'm in your hands, and you're going to help me through this."*
>
> —STEPHANIE

It is perhaps unsurprising that women identified trust as important to a good birth—that having a trusting relationship with their midwife or doctor was part of what made women feel secure and part of what made their birth good.

Of course, trust is a piece of how we relate to health care providers, into which I delve deeply in Chapter 4. But it's also important to understand how trust contributes to our sense of security specifically, and how its absence makes us feel vulnerable to threat.

If the need for trust in birth is unsurprising, I think the emphasis on trust is in fact remarkable. For much of what women have to read about birth these days urges distrust, especially of doctors and midwives who work in hospital settings. For instance, in her recent book *Pushed* and on her website, journalist Jennifer Block depicts contemporary birth as potentially and often unavoidably adversarial: be on your guard, she advises, in order to avoid medical interventions and what she calls a "pushed" birth. If you can't give birth at home, urges Block, find other ways to push back: *avoid* interventions, *negotiate* birth positions, and *refuse* episiotomy. This hardly sounds like the stuff of a relationship built on trust.

To some degree, Block is right in her admonition that we must choose providers carefully, that we must not trust blindly. She is right that some in the business of birth will not have our best interests in mind, and it's well worth figuring out who those people are and protecting ourselves from them if possible. But two major fallacies undergird Block's view and leave women feeling disappointed and misled. The first is that we can predict whether a provider is trustworthy or not based on how or where she practices, and we can't. To the extent that it is overly skeptical (and I think it is) to regard with suspicion any hospital-based provider, it is naive to blindly trust a provider who practices out of the home. Credentials can tell us just so much; then we need to look deeper.

But there is a second and perhaps more important fallacy: that we can somehow dispense with trust in birth and we'll be okay; that the good birth these days is about putting up a good fight. For some this might be the case, but I would offer that they are the fortunate few who dodge the twists and turns in birth that demand we trust if we are to feel personally secure. If birth advocacy like Block's has helped to raise awareness and carve out room for low-intervention births, its sometimes vitriolic nature can lead us to neglect our need for security during our transition to motherhood. More often than not—and no matter where it is done—birth is marked by uncertainty, and navigating such requires we trust those around us; we are in their hands, we rely on their assurances, and we want to feel that they are on our side. Birth is one of those times in life where we need others' help. We have no choice but to allow other people in, give them the power to help or harm, to indelibly shift the trajectory of our lives. And so we must trust them. For in the absence of trust, giving birth can feel like clinging to a tightrope strung across a deep ravine.

It felt that way for Danielle, a woman I met recently while I was visiting New York. She worked for a publishing house—was brilliant, savvy, a hard-hitting feminist, and mother of two-year-old Callum. Before his birth, she read the latest books and blogs, and on the basis of those went into birth with the sense that she'd have to fight for the sort of birth she wanted: a low-intervention birth in a hospital setting. "I think home birth is irresponsible," she told me, "but I certainly didn't want to be strapped to a hospital bed and given medications I didn't need." So she hired a doula to "run interference" and found an obstetrics group in town with a reasonable reputation and doctors she believed were competent, if not exactly congenial. Let's just say she didn't particularly trust them, but it didn't strike her that she needed to; not, at least, until minutes after Callum was born and Danielle found herself out on that tightrope.

With new baby in arms, Danielle realized all was not well—she was bleeding heavily. Her nurse moved to give her medication; her doula resisted. The doctor arrived and urged her to accept a pill that would make the bleeding stop; the doula urged her not to take the pill, emphasizing its risks. Holding her baby, blood gushing between her legs, Danielle was scared and stuck, trapped between dissenting providers. Up to that point, she'd felt great about holding her ground; but now what she wanted—needed—more than anything else was to share that space with someone she knew had her best interests in mind. Someone she could trust. But the bickering doctor and doula appeared oriented toward their respective agendas; she couldn't tell who had her health in mind, whom she could trust. Ultimately, the bleeding did stop, without medication, but Danielle ended up with a transfusion and a bottle of constipating iron pills before all was said and done. Even two years later, she was flummoxed by the challenge that birth presented: "How would I ever know," she asked me, "in a moment like that, who was right?"

Indeed, how can we know? Birth will bring unexpected challenges we can't navigate on our own. We must rely on the knowledge and goodwill of others for our safety; we cannot give birth single-handedly. Trust is key.

I realize this sounds simple, but it's not. Having people you trust around you is as important to security as access to lifesaving equipment, comfortable and private surroundings, and a calm atmosphere—maybe more so. This was the lesson for Liz in her second birth. She knew from the first time around that, for her, feeling safe and secure in birth depended on being in a structured hospital environment. All of that was in place. But once there, her trust was betrayed, and nothing could make her feel safe after that.

In Chapter 1, I talked at some length about Liz's second birth, wherein she asked for an epidural and was assured that the anesthesiologist was "on his way," only to have to wait for hours, until she was too far along for his help. But what I didn't cover in Chapter 1 is that what was lost for Liz was something more important to her than the anesthetized labor she'd planned on; it was trust in those around her. Liz ultimately realized the true cost of broken trust in a riveting moment of uncertainty in birth, after her daughter was born and she wasn't sure all was well. Now that she had lost trust in her providers, their reassurances—critical to her sense of safety—were no longer meaningful.

> I pushed like twice, and baby came out, the cord was wrapped around her neck . . . No crying, no nothing. I'm lying there, I'm thinking, "What's happening?" I said, "Is she okay?" Everyone's telling me, "Yes, she'll be fine, she'll be fine." I don't *trust* anybody at this point because . . . I didn't feel like I had been monitored very closely and I felt like no one was really being up front with me the whole time.
>
> I looked over. I could see [the pediatrics team] bagging her [giving her oxygen] . . . Everyone kept telling me, "She'll be fine. This is pretty common that this happens. She'll be fine." Thank God, after a minute or two, which seemed like ten minutes or more to me . . . she was crying and everything was okay and I was able to hold her.

As is often the case with trust, its necessity emerges most vividly when it is betrayed. Liz couldn't take any assurance to heart—she'd lost trust in her providers when they had failed to come through on their promises about her epidural, and now their words fell flat. She needed tangible proof to press back a sense of impending disaster; only her newborn daughter's cry would do. Until the sweet screech came forth, broken trust meant that, for Liz, personal security was out of reach.

Liz went into birth trusting her provider and felt the sting of trust when it was lost. Many other women we talked to in anticipation of birth were less trusting at the outset and thought that having a good birth would require a fight, that it was naive to think they could trust their doctor, or that trust was nice but not necessary. But when women looked back on their births, they realized how important it was to trust if they were to feel safe and secure, and how important safety and security were to having a good birth.

Such comes through when we compare the experiences of Carol and Lara. Both planned home births; both ended up being transferred to the hospital for medical reasons. But while Carol felt her birth was still good, Lara assessed hers as nothing short of traumatic.

When we met her, Carol was pregnant for the first time. A tiny-framed, university-based scientist, she'd combed through the studies on safety in birth, thought about what she valued, and decided on home birth. Then she found a midwife she adored and, perhaps more important, trusted.

Mid-labor, at home, the midwife checked her and realized that her baby was coming out bottom first (breech). She told Carol they needed to transfer her to the hospital, and called an ambulance. Carol told us:

> I felt okay. I wasn't scared. My husband was scared. But I felt fine. And [the midwife] was able to go in the ambulance with me . . . and she kind of coached me through the whole eight-minute drive to the hospital.

Carol said her feelings of security, of not being scared, were "a big part of" why her experience was good. When we asked her why she didn't feel scared, even in her situation, she pointed to her midwife and the plans they'd made together, to their strong and trusting relationship.

We had a concrete course of action—I'm close to the hospital, so things were in place. No one was saying, "Oh my gosh, you're going to die!" They were just saying, "This is happening, we're changing plans, here's what we're going to do, we're going to help you through it, and baby's fine."

In contrast to Carol, Lara's transfer experience was harrowing. After laboring all day and pushing for two hours, she started passing thick meconium, indicating the baby was stressed. Her midwife encouraged her to continue laboring at home, but eventually Lara decided herself that it was time to go to the hospital. For lack of planning, her husband was at the wheel, and Lara endured more than an hour's uncertainty in transit to the hospital:

I was like, "Just get it out." [My husband] was driving. We should have had another plan. My midwife was in the back of her van with me. There was no cushion, there were no blankets; all she did was grab her bags and her oxygen and threw [them] in the back of her van and we were on our way. We got lost. We got stuck in a traffic jam. It took us over an hour to get to the hospital. I thought I was dying. I was screaming like a primal scream. It wasn't even like an "ow." It was like, "Aaaahhhh," screaming. I was scared to death.

Part of what differentiated Lara's and Carol's experiences involved having—or not having—plans in place if they needed to go to the hospital. But talking through those contingencies requires a certain honesty and openness—willingness to concede that the hoped-for birth will be strived for but cannot be guaranteed—with trust no doubt helping that conversation along. When Lara looked back on the birth, it wasn't about traffic or the unpadded surface of the van; it was about the trust lacking between her and her midwife. And it wasn't just sour grapes. If the lack of trustworthiness came into sharp relief in retrospect, it didn't feel surprising to Lara, who pressed away a creeping suspicion throughout pregnancy that something was missing.

I always felt like I was an inconvenience to my midwife. I didn't click with her at all. And we got that sense from day one. But she was the only one that could do home birth that I knew of at that time . . . I knew in my heart she was not [great], and I always felt uncomfortable. I never felt I could be myself with her. I knew it wasn't right, but I didn't care because I was going to have my baby at home and it was only a short time. It was like one day, two days at most I had to be with her. And I could do it.

Yes, birth is only a day, only an hour, but the fact of the matter is that a good birth depends not on getting the birth you want, but feeling safe and secure in the process. Without trust, personal security—and possibly, a good birth—will elude us.

Finding Personal Security in Birth

As I thought about Pam—my patient who moved to Minnesota and called me mid-pregnancy—in the weeks leading up to her birth, I worried about her. She'd given birth three times before, in the hospital, with me. But it wasn't like she was going to get on a plane and find her way back to that space she and I knew we could forge. She needed to find a new safe space in Minnesota.

One way to think about it (and my first conclusion regarding her) was that she should get out of Dodge—that we obstetricians and our knives are the pressing threat for women and that people like Pam should stay home to give birth. Lots of women (like Maisie) reason this way and decide on home birth just because home feels like the safest place to bring a baby into the world.

The other way to think about it—and I think the correct way—is that it is not just about obstetricians and knives and steering clear of us. It's about finding *personal security* in birth, in the deepest sense of the word. Pam needed to think about what it was that would make her feel secure. For her that meant being in a hospital, with ready access to technology, even if that closeness invited risk of technology's overreach. It also meant creating a space that felt calm, private, and comfortable.

But perhaps most important, she needed to make sure the person caring for her had her best interests in mind—was a person worthy of her trust. It was probably worth her considering why she felt she needed to call me: Did she just want some information or comfort, or was it about a wobbling belief that she was in trustworthy hands? I cannot say whether the doctor who delivered Sebastian fit the bill. Pam did end up with a cesarean for another ten-pound baby. She and Sebastian emerged as healthy as could be, and she was fine with the surgery, which gave her an excuse for a few weeks to sit in a comfy glider with her baby rather than manage her brood. I cannot say whether her cesarean was the key to averted disaster or evidence that her doctor lost his nerve, and I'll never know. But it is really Pam who will live with the questions, or not. It is Pam for whom the remains of the day might be niggling worries about the necessity of cesarean, or certainty that—by virtue of trust—surgical birth was lifesaving and just as full of sweetness and sanctity as the vaginal births that preceded it. I can't say I've talked to Pam about this, but she sends me a Christmas card every year, plastered with smiles of her children wrapping their arms around one another. My hope, of course, is that she can honestly share with each a birth story that she holds dear.

Birth is a threshold; it marks our entry into motherhood and our baby's entry into the world. And thresholds, it turns out, are special places that cultivate particular sorts of behaviors—and a certain level of fear—in human beings.

According to anthropologist Mary Douglas, the in-between states make us anxious; they emerge as threatening. In the order of the world, they are spaces of disarray. "Though we seek to create order," she tells us, "we do not simply condemn disorder. We recognize that it is destructive to existing patterns; also that it has potentiality. It symbolizes both danger and power." And so pregnancy and birth, often breathtakingly powerful and (now) safe by modern standards, may always strike us as dangerous. It is perhaps, then, no wonder that women strive for a sense of security in the face of such a monumental event.

For as women tell us, birth—whatever the venue—is replete with dangers. Some of those dangers involve very small risks of very rare things that we dread. Some of those dangers stem from the interventions aimed at their elimination. Some dangers stem from potential harms of violation—of the body, of relationships, of sacred space. And some stem from the threat of abandonment during a time of need. Women also tell us that a good birth requires crafting an approach that makes them feel personally secure amid the things that emerge as threatening.

The challenge will continue to be cultivating that security. Where it won't be found is in insisting on the safety of the event, or dismissing its dangers, physical and otherwise, or imagining we have the means to eliminate them. "Dangers," Douglas reminds us, "are manifold and omnipresent." In birth, whether realized or not, they shape our notion of the good.

What does this mean for those of you facing delivery? My view is that while you need not dwell on the risks of birthing, don't turn away from them either, or pretend they somehow don't exist. A good birth depends on engaging with them, understanding which risks loom largest for you, and crafting an approach that keeps them, realistically, at a comfortable distance. And, the wise women of the Good Birth Project tell us, safety doesn't reside simply in stark choices like home or hospital, but in the highly personal and particular understanding of the "security trio" of comfort, privacy, and calmness. Ask your friends, your mom, people you love and trust, what worked for them, what surprised them, what they ended up needing to feel safe and secure, keeping in mind that feelings of security are built on a lifetime of experiences and so your trio will be unique. As such, finding personal security in birth will be a process, will require a look inside as well as due diligence on the topic of maternity care options. Consider keeping a journal—writing things down to get a sense of your hopes and fears. Putting things down on paper can be a helpful means to understand and, yes, contain in some way things that can feel massive or unmanageable in the absence of words. It has certainly helped me.

Finally, a certain degree of openness to help is simply vital—from friends, family, health care providers. As I approached my fourth cesarean, you might think I would have had it all figured out, that I would feel certain, would have a well-worn route to personal security for myself in birth. Not so—and a good friend of mine (who was also once my patient) sensed it one day as we gabbed on our way in to work. A fan of hypnosis for birth, she offered me a set of CDs to listen to in preparation for Will's delivery. I found them to be a source of comfort and reassurance, a new and powerful tool to help me manage persistent fears as I headed toward surgery. If I hadn't been open—genuinely open—to an approach about which I knew a fair amount, I might never have had that incredibly valuable source of comfort that made such a difference to me. (Indeed, that friend who offered it used it herself in all her births, including the one I attended, and I've referred many a patient to a favorite hypnosis instructor in town.)

Finally, do your best to disentangle from the birth wars—birth is no place to do battle; avoid it if you can. Surround yourself with people—including your health care provider—whom you like and, more to the point, trust, who make you feel safe and secure. For despite its dangers, birth is at its best a place for partnership and peace.

four

Connectedness

Here, under my heart
you'll keep
till it's time
for us to meet,
& we come apart
that we may come
together,
& you are born
remembering
the wavesound
of my blood,
the thunder of my heart,
& like your mother
always dreaming
of the sea.

—ERICA JONG, "THE BIRTH OF THE WATER BABY"

It is often said in medicine that the cleanliness of an office correlates inversely with the brilliance of a doctor. If that's the case, I'm married to a genius, and fortunately Kim and I both can tolerate material chaos. Yet in the midst of the stacks of unread mail, journal articles, and our children's artwork, there was one piece of paper that stayed on the floor too long.

At some point during the days following our son Will's arrival, Kim pressed the "Print" button on his phone and transmitted to our unreliable printer a photo he took of me holding William, just two hours after his birth.

The photo must have printed in Kim's absence and fluttered to the floor, where it landed faceup. It depicted one of our "first moments"—Will was at last in my arms, both of us tethered to IVs but feeling temporarily oblivious to our surroundings in the neonatal intensive care unit. It is a moment I will never forget, both in its initial sweetness and stark brevity.

For a while, brevity stole the stage. Minutes after the photo was taken, a resident approached me with a thick binder, a pen, and a request for my signature. The proximity of my cesarean meant I was in a wheelchair; it faced the wall, so I had to crane my neck to see the bright-eyed young man in scrubs. There was a consent form in his hands—a long one, full of paragraphs about which I knew too much, describing unlikely complications I now found unimaginable.

The moment was one that I had in some ways anticipated over the course of my pregnancy. Midway through it, an ultrasound found a mysterious elliptical mass inside William's belly that had the sonographers and obstetricians, the smartest people we knew, scratching their heads. Ultimately it meant a pre-birth consultation with a pediatric surgeon, who recommended that we take more pictures of the offending mass after birth. Innocent enough, but he wanted to do it on William's first day, in his first hours. The surgeon wanted to make sure he was in town, in case they had to operate.

At the time the photo was taken, we were in the midst of his plan. His minion, the resident, told me that William's IV wasn't working well and that they wanted to put an intravenous line through his freshly cut umbilical cord. The line would find its end point in the vena cava (the large vessel that takes blood back to the heart). It would be easier to manage and unlikely to come out or get clogged. I realized that he was proposing a central line, which, despite my postpartum haze, I knew had risks that were far from trivial.

Kim and I ultimately declined (they found a vein in Will's other arm), though we had to put up a fight and then endure, for the time being, a label of "difficult" parents. The label was tolerable if less than ideal. What felt intolerable to me, though, was something lost in the process—my first moments with Will were interrupted, and I'd never get them back.

So for weeks that picture sat on the floor of Kim's office. I'd walk by it, or over it, often with Will in arms, on my way to the bathroom or to find something in the office piles. Until one day, finally, I stopped stepping over it. I picked it up and saw sweetness instead of brevity. That moment wasn't what I had envisioned, it wasn't my ideal—but it was mine, ours. A rocky start, but the beginning of our life together, and for that reason something to hold on to—and perhaps, eventually, to celebrate.

Connectedness in Birth

At first blush it may seem obvious—of course women want and need to feel connected to others in birth. When I was just starting the project, I was discussing it at a dinner party with Ben, a friend of mine from medical school. He recalled the "saddest moment" of his rotation in obstetrics: when he caught the baby of a woman who came to the hospital unaccompanied—no mom, no spouse, and nobody on their way. She labored alone, gave birth alone. Just she and Ben and a couple of nurses were there to bear witness— and once he'd handed her the swaddled infant, he headed to the cafeteria and cried.

Ben—if a sensitive guy—is no sap. Indeed, his intuitions about connectedness in birth are reflected across the spectrum of providers and the public. Women are flooded with advice about finding the right "support" person in birth; a number of books discuss the advantages of getting a "trained labor companion" or doula. Midwifery is famous for its distinguishing etymology— *midwife* literally means "with woman." Fathers (as well as other loved ones) have entered the delivery room, and almost everyone considers the end of the smoky-waiting-room era a hugely positive advance in maternity care. And finally, there is the emphasis on "bonding" with the baby, and the ever-contested notion of mother-baby "attachment" that some (controversially) claim is indelibly shaped by our babies' first moments outside.

In giving birth to Will, I felt something that I always knew to be the case, though perhaps had struggled to put into words: that birth both intensifies and strains our sense of connectedness. Indeed, the possibility of being—or feeling—alone in birth, as in death, is a nearly universal source of dread; its realization is often experienced or recollected with profound regret. And the need to feel connected came through in story after story told to us by women of the Good Birth Project.

Yet if the importance of connectedness is obvious, why it's important and how to meaningfully achieve it are less clear. This is where women's voices come in.

What we heard from the women in the Good Birth Project is that a good birth is indeed one in which we feel connected—to our spouse or partner, our loved ones, our health care providers, and perhaps most important, our babies. But if connectedness is a complicated matter in daily life, birth brings its challenges to the forefront. For instance, women speak of needing a certain kind of intimate support in birth. As in all intimacies, it's about having the *right* person there—the right doctor or midwife, spouse, parent, or friend. No doubt, we can be surrounded by people and feel alone, or we can be with one person and feel deeply, completely accompanied.

Take mother of two Molly, who devastatingly lost a set of twins the first time she gave birth. They came early—way too early for doctors to do anything to save their lives. Afterward, her husband had to slip out to feed the dogs (and I imagine regain his footing in the world), and so, she recalls, she was left alone in the hospital for several hours. She explains:

> A nurse or somebody probably told the chaplain at the hospital that I was alone, because somebody suddenly shows up. And that was awkward . . . he didn't really know what to say to me. He did his best. But I felt like I had to put him at ease in his discomfort over his awkwardness over it. I think at that point I would have preferred to have been left alone.

Of course, people often fumble and fail in attempts to accompany someone in the midst of a loss, and the same is true in the case of birth, even of a healthy child. People don't know what to say, don't know when to stay or go. In fact, I experienced as much when I was in labor with my first child, Grant. Kim had decided to work through rather than cancel his full morning of surgery, about which I tried not to be infuriated. In his attempts to assuage that fury, he sent one of his close work colleagues—whom I knew pretty well—to keep me company while I labored and he was scrubbed. But after about fifteen minutes, I realized I wanted nothing more than for her to leave, and fortunately my mom arrived and the ill-considered companion made herself scarce. She was a perfectly nice person, but a stranger in intimate space. Feeling accompanied in birth means that the right people—and only the right people—are with us: people who will support us without needing reciprocal care, people who will make us feel accompanied without the attention from us that less-than-intimate company usually requires.

But in birth, feeling accompanied is no simple matter. Intimate relationships are in flux—families of two become families of three, women become mothers and men become fathers, our mothers and fathers become grandparents. In addition, since we need help bringing our children into the world, we must let others into intimate spaces—doctors, midwives, nurses, doulas, some of whom we will have chosen, will have had a chance to get to know; others may be strangers. Finally, birth is about our babies, our children, and our relationship to them. For some of us, birth feels like a beginning, for others a separation, and for others still a seismic shift in the way we relate to the person who has inhabited our body for the preceding several months.

In this chapter, I turn to women's thoughts on connectedness and ways in which they negotiate and understand their relationships to others—health care providers, friends and family, the baby—during birth. Many will find riveting moments experienced or lost, opportunities to forge and shape relationships as we bring babies into the world. It turns out that those moments are as different as the babies we bear, rarely as envisioned, sometimes disappointing, and other times beyond what we could have imagined. If moments are important, women tell us there is much more at stake; relationships that begin or change during delivery go on and on outside the birthing suite. And as relationships start, end, and evolve, birth moves all too many of us to consider not just how and to whom we are connected, but deep existential questions about the degree to which we are, or are not, alone.

Connecting to Baby

For nine months, you just wait. Even the time before you get pregnant, you still are thinking about it. You just wait and wait and all you want to do is hold that baby. To see him so close but so far away, and not know when they're going to give him to you—that was hard. And it really didn't take that long, but I just remember waiting was hard. After the labor and the birth, it just felt like I deserved to hold that baby.

—NAOMI

One of the first women we interviewed for the Good Birth Project was Tonya, mother of two young boys, Darrell and Isaiah. Compared with Darrell's birth, she told us, Isaiah's—a planned cesarean—was pretty wonderful. Darrell had arrived amid the chaos of an emergency, a bleeding vessel in the edge of the placenta, which demanded immediate surgical delivery. The worst part, Tonya told us, was that right after he was born, she didn't get to see him. "I didn't get to see, touch, feel him or anything after having him. They whisked him away and there was nothing I could do about it." After the pediatrics team wheeled the bassinet out of the operating room, her father scurried down the hallway after it and snapped pictures of his grandson with a digital camera. "I saw Darrell's picture," Tonya told us, "before I ever saw him in person."

No doubt, the experience has had an enduring sting. Even though she had a chance to hold Darrell in the intensive care nursery the day after his birth, it was a full two weeks before she felt "that connect"—when they were home, at last, together. "He's my sweet, the light of my life now," she told me. "But I've always felt like I missed something, like something I should have had is gone."

In dozens of interviews after Tonya's, we heard the same thing—that what is critical to a good birth is being, feeling, connected to baby.

It wasn't a surprise. Far from it. In fact, I knew it long before I had any children of my own, long before I set foot on Labor and Delivery, before I attended medical school for that matter. What I knew of birth before my medical training was the comparisons my parents would make between my entry into the world and that of my older brother, which I alluded to in the

Introduction—a story that has been told and retold: he, born in Washington, D.C.'s posh Sibley Hospital, dragged out of my sedated mother with forceps, my father confined to a smoky waiting room; I, born two years later at Stanford without anesthesia or offending instruments, placed immediately on my mother's belly, to her and my father's immediate and long-standing delight. Mine was the good birth, no doubt, and that first moment in my mother's arms its unquestioned high point.

But it's a high point that depends on so many things going right—out of the question for Tonya in her first birth and seemingly out of reach for so many other women, for so many reasons. Advances in maternity care have improved matters, including efforts to get mom and baby together in the first hour after birth and keep them together as much as possible after that. But physiology and fate as well as insensitive practitioners and outdated practices can get in the way, leaving too many to wonder: If the good birth requires that immediate, slippery skin-to-skin union, might a good birth, realistically, be out of reach?

The short answer is no. If the women of the Good Birth Project endorse the notion that connectedness to baby is important, they also tell us there are many ways to get it—it is not a door that opens and closes, and for some women it's better delayed, if slightly. As we look deeper into connecting to the baby, you'll see that what we need to do is press aside a romanticized and narrow story that has captured our gaze, and recognize the myriad ways women connect, and connect well, en route to a good birth.

For many women, that initial connection is wonderful, even if it doesn't happen the moment of delivery, and even if it doesn't happen exactly the way the mom had planned. Remember Mara from Chapter 3, whose first delivery was an emergency cesarean: she was surprised how connected she felt to her son Jacob after his frightening entry. If relief was the initial emotion, there was a moment afterward that Mara told us was "one of the highlights of my life so far." As soon as she rolled into the recovery room, she got to hold him. For Mara, who'd envisioned a drug-free labor and the moments-old baby put on her chest, you might think there would be some regret, but not so. "I couldn't sit up, because I had the epidural in, so they just put him in the crook of my arm, and he was just nuzzled in." Not what she expected, but "just a really perfect experience."

Going through the cesarean made Mara reexamine her thoughts about them. "I thought they were kind of cold procedures because the mom doesn't get to hold the baby right away. I just thought they would take the baby out and put it under lights in the corner . . . But having gone through it now, I think it's probably just as nice." No doubt, cesareans can be cold procedures. The point is that they don't have to be. Moments to connect are often there—you just have to look a little harder to find them sometimes (and we doctors need to work harder to cultivate them).

Many (including Mara) think that if we can safely avoid cesarean, by all means we should, for all sorts of reasons—more opportunities for connectedness being just one of them. But delivering vaginally doesn't guarantee that you'll feel connected to your baby in those first moments either.

Lots of books on birth will tell you the problem is medication during labor—that it makes you too groggy to be able to connect to your baby right away. And to some extent this is true. Liz recollected that, in the moments after she delivered her first, with no epidural and just one dose of IV medication, "I was so drugged up that I couldn't even see her. I had to close one eye to focus, because I was just so loopy I was like, 'I can't even see my baby! I literally cannot see straight!'"

Feeling the way Liz did can get in the way of presence and bearing witness, which I talked about in Chapter 2: the cloudiness of being medicated can interfere with women's sense that they've been the deliverer, that they were the ones giving birth. But some women also told us how feeling loopy from medication interfered with something else that they valued deeply, namely their ability to forge that initial connection with baby.

Does this mean that to feel connected to baby you have to go drug-free? According to the women of the Good Birth Project, that doesn't necessarily make the difference. Some women found that pain and exhaustion can be just as distracting. For instance, Natalie reflected on her first moments after delivering vaginally, without anesthesia: "I was surprised. I wanted and expected to have that initial feeling when she was born, to be like, 'Oh my God, I'm in love with this baby.' But I didn't, not right away." Natalie was tired—exhausted, in fact. She'd had a long labor, had pushed for four hours, and delivered with a vacuum. "When she finally came out," reflected Natalie, "I honestly cried because I was so relieved to be done. I mean, I can't emphasize enough that that is what I was celebrating. You know, the baby was totally secondary to being done, it was so hard."

There are certainly plenty of women who feel instantly connected when they deliver without medications—their birth stories are the ones that get posted in blogs and construed as ideals in countless books promoting "natural birth." But theirs is not the only road to connectedness, and there are many ways to that connectedness that women say is so important. Indeed, there is more than one way to connect with baby; wanting to do so doesn't limit you to one sort of birth, and it doesn't mean that you have to deliver without anesthesia. In fact, enhanced connectedness between mom and baby is the reason some women value their cesareans, the reason some seasoned midwives argue for better anesthetic options, and the reason some women choose epidurals in the first place.

Indeed, connection was the very reason Liz was so dead set on an epidural for her second birth. She didn't want to feel loopy, the way the IV meds had made her feel, or to have to depend on pictures snapped to recollect her first moments with her baby. As she approached her second birth, she told us, "I was thinking, I'd really like to, after she comes out, be in the moment. And thankfully I was able to. I was mentally very clearheaded—just numb from the waist down." And though parts of that birth were rough, the first moments after her daughter arrived were just what she had hoped for. "That experience of the second was better, because it was so emotional when she started crying . . . to see her, and feel very connected to her."

In fact, connectedness runs right through arguments made for expanding women's options to different kinds of anesthesia. Revered nurse-midwife Judith Rooks has for years championed making nitrous oxide available to women in labor. For exhausted moms who don't want an epidural, it can take the edge off—help them to rest and gather strength. But it can be put away and its effects leave a woman's system in five minutes, so that when she delivers, she can connect with her infant, exhaustion helpfully pressed aside, her mind unclouded by medication.

Beyond decisions around medication, there are several more points to be made about connecting to your baby in birth. First is simply that the hour immediately after a baby is born isn't always the right time to connect, even when the two of you are together and nothing seems to be in your way. In other words, a good birth doesn't—or at least shouldn't—depend on how that hour goes. The second is that connection with baby has much to do with what else is going on in the woman's life. And the third is that, by its very nature, birth is as much a letting go of something as it is the beginning of something new; this can also affect how connecting with baby unfolds for us moms. Let's take these points one at a time.

Many of us get fixated on the first hour after birth, and understandably so. It's come to hold a nearly magical aura in the past few decades, following an article published in the prestigious *New England Journal of Medicine* in 1972. Its authors, pediatrician-neonatologist team John Kennell and Marshall Klaus, postulated a "sensitive period"—a period right after birth when the cement that glues moms and babies together is best poured—or so it is claimed. The two built a career on the topic of maternal-infant attachment, and they've been honored by many organizations that champion "family-friendly" birth practices. Their efforts have certainly moved maternity care practices in the right direction, but the impact has not been entirely positive.

The problem is that hour's magical status. In that hour, if things don't happen a certain way, don't feel a certain way, then worries creep in that there is something wrong, that we have failed somehow, that our relationship with our child is forever altered, and for the worse.

Now I can tell you that the data are soft, and that follow-up studies have had conflicting results. Even advocates of the view would counter that the first hour is a "sensitive" period, not a "critical" period. But it's a hard sell for new mothers to distinguish the two, and moms have the tendency to wonder despite objective evidence and heartfelt reassurances.

Take Katha, whose baby was diagnosed with a heart condition that would require surgery right after birth in a hospital in a distant city. "Going in," she told us, "I felt okay." But then, she reflects, birth was a "roller coaster" and her inability to connect with her baby right away an enduring source of guilt.

> The emotional connection that you normally have when you first have a baby—I didn't get that till like five days later. I didn't hold him until we got to [the other city]. I was sort of discon-nected from him for a while, even the first night, because I had just had the C-section. I went to see him in the NICU, but I was

pretty weak and I had to sit in a wheelchair, and it was very, very uncomfortable. So I needed to lie down. I couldn't physically sit there all night with him. I felt very guilty. I felt like a horrible mother because I couldn't stay there.

I will tell you that Katha and many women like her do connect with their children as time goes on. If they worry that something was lost, those worries eventually get pressed aside by the certainty that they do love their child, and love them deeply—by the certainty that whatever opportunities were missed in the process are not the whole. They look to their days of mothering and conclude, as did *New York Times* journalist Samantha Shapiro, writing about her "natural birth" that went by the wayside, "Eight months with my son have offered ample evidence that there is not only one opportunity for joy."

No doubt Shapiro is right, that mothering brings solace and wisdom, assurance that deep connection happens over time. But I don't think that means we have to or even should retire our hopes about birth, for finding the good *in* it, rather than *after* it.

Indeed, experienced moms tell us that that first hour isn't the only time for magic. More to the point, it isn't always the right time for it. For instance, Christina told us that though given the opportunity, she didn't *want* to hold her baby right away.

I heard the cry. And I was shaking, and I felt very unsettled. It wasn't joy. It was relief, tremendous relief having that baby out of me. But I was shaking and I didn't want my baby to feel my shaking. So I didn't hold her right away. And I think the nurse thought there was something wrong with me. But really, for my first experience with [my daughter], I didn't want her to feel me shaking. I wanted her to feel me strong.

But the moment came when she was ready:

I remember, when I first nursed her, she latched on right away, and she looked me straight in the eye. And you know, they say babies don't do that, but she looked me straight in the eye and it made such a difference to me.

Many women, in fact, said love came later—just a little later. For instance, Natalie, who like Christina felt only relief when her first daughter was born, said their "defining moment" was hours after. As she puts it:

> I went back to the room and I went to sleep, and then at midnight the light comes in from nowhere, and it's the door opening to my room. The nurse wheels her in, and then I started crying. I was like, "Oh my God, there's my baby. I'm a mother."

Or Leslie, who gave birth twice in birth centers and once at home. Reflecting on that first hour, she told us:

> I have to say, that first hour I don't feel like myself. I just want to roll up in a ball and cry. You see these videos of women who are so elated—how come it's not like that for me? I don't have these goo-goo, ga-ga feelings the first time I see my babies. And I feel guilty.

But like several other women in the Good Birth Project, she told us she comes around after an hour or so, when she does feel like herself again. "By then," she tells us, "I'm just as emotional but am thinking, 'I can't believe God gave me this perfect gift,' and I just want to nurse him and not let anyone else hold him." But after three births, she's come to accept that just takes a while.

Mother of three Candace had quick vaginal deliveries. She told us that it was nice to see the baby right away and have the "moment of realizing that the baby is actually here, and getting to see what they looked like." But she appreciated that the baby was taken away to do vital signs.

> I just needed that short moment, and that was fine. I wanted to have some time to [decompress] from birth, unwind, have a moment to get cleaned up. I wanted to get into a clean gown, clean sheets, not have to be sitting in the same spot where I just delivered.

Midwife Bev told us of that after an intense labor with her second, she also needed to recoup.

> I pushed her out and I fell forward and they were saying, "Do you want to see the baby?" And I didn't know. I'm like, I need to catch my grip. Because I was grunting like a bull—I mean, they were trying to talk to me and I couldn't hear their words. So it wasn't so much that I had this totally granola experience of the baby coming and immediately being on my chest . . . It wasn't sort of the intimate bonding with my baby.

Women should not feel pressured to make the bonding immediate and strong. There is a time and place for connecting, a way of feeling, and it often doesn't happen during that first hour. The connection will come when the time is right and you're ready for it.

The same point could be made about rooming in, wherein mom and baby share a room for the duration of their hospital stay. Rooming in has become more the norm after Klaus and Kennell. There are many women—myself included—who are happy about the shift to keeping babies and moms in the same postpartum room rather than wheeling babies off to the nursery (in fact, the full-term nursery where I trained in obstetrics was moved in the past decade from a generous, light-filled space to what was once a broom closet, rarely graced by newborns, who now stay with their mothers). But it's not the ideal or preferred situation for everyone—far from it. My obstetrician made fun of me when I complained that I hadn't slept all night because Will was in the intensive care unit instead of in my room, and I was missing out on that intimate time I'd anticipated we would share in the hospital. "Most people complain," she said, with a twinkle in her eye, "that they haven't slept all night because their babies *are* in the room."

The fact is, though, in the days after labor, we all need time to regroup and get ready for the rest of our lives as mothers. Lots of women need a real break—some solid sleep, a good shower or two, if we are going to be able to handle the days ahead. We need to get to feeling like ourselves again. But with the rooming-in mantra so often linked with attachment and, more controversially, good motherhood, asking for a little peace gets dicey and invites all manner of judgment. Dare we say that those days of long postpartum stays—when nurses helped care for baby, covered beds with crisp sheets and hospital corners, and delivered decent meals on trays—don't sound *all* bad? The truth is that some women rest better with their baby nearby; others appreciate resting assured that competent care is being provided down the hall. And those of us who have been through it a time or two know that there will be plenty of one-on-one time in the days ahead, so getting a break in the hospital is just getting while the getting is good.

This brings me to the second point about connecting to baby that I think often gets missed. It doesn't just depend on how you deliver or the way in which you and your baby meet, but what's going on in your life beyond the labor suite—and you have to take stock of that when you are thinking about your birth and how you feel about it, as should those who are helping you through.

Take mother of two Simone. Her pregnancy had been uncomplicated, but near term she stopped being able to feel her baby move. She ended up at the hospital, where the doctors were worried enough to recommend inducing labor. A hairsbreadth away from a cesarean, she delivered vaginally—amid a swarm of pediatricians—her healthy daughter. "I remember pushing, pushing, pushing, her delivering with forceps, basically getting this picture of her being okay, and then kind of crashing. I don't remember when she left, or how long she was gone—maybe an hour, maybe more."

It was a scary birth for Simone, though she was attended by doctors she trusted, and ended up, for all intents and purposes, physically unscathed. Looking back on that birth, though, one thing continues to rivet her gaze. "I do still wonder," she confided, "if that [lost hour] affected the bonding." Simone had a tough postpartum course and suffered through what sounds to me like postpartum depression—days filled with darkness and more pointedly a "complete disconnect" from the "little bundle that I'd waited for all my life." Having missed that crucial hour, she wondered, would there be any way to make up for lost time?

I'd remind Simone to look beyond that hour—not just because it's sensitive (if we believe that it is—and remember, it's controversial), but because so much else is relevant. For instance, Simone also told us that her grandmother, who was very close to her, had a stroke within hours of the birth. "It was a hard time in my life," Simone told us through tears, "because I was really looking forward to sharing it with my grandmother, and she wasn't there . . . That, for me, was the first real loss in my life." To be sure, it can be hard to forge a new connection when you are losing someone whom you have always loved.

Finally, it's important to remember that delivery is preceded by pregnancy—and how we experienced being pregnant makes a difference to how delivering a baby feels to a new mother. For the outside observer, birth is when a baby arrives—when we finally get to feast our eyes on the newest member of a family and welcome a new person into our midst. But some of us also feel, in birth, our baby's departure. This can be particularly true for those who feel connected to their babies (or fetuses, depending on whom you ask) *before* delivery. It's not like they arrive on a doorstep—they've been around, so to speak, for a while.

When I was in residency, I recall feeling envious of a young and pregnant faculty member who gracefully toted her belly around the wards. After rounds, she would often say something like "All right, if everything is okay here on Labor and Delivery, Lacy and I will be in the call room"—Lacy being the name she'd settled on for the child she was expecting. And then she'd spin around and proceed down the hallway by herself—sort of.

Perhaps it was just a sassy quip—for which my colleague was famous—but the sense that in pregnancy we are accompanied in some very substantive way is hardly far-fetched. As my friend Maggie Little once wrote in a philosophy article:

> To be pregnant is to be *inhabited*. It is to be *occupied*. It is to be in a state of physical intimacy of a particularly thoroughgoing nature. The fetus intrudes on the body massively; whatever medical risks one faces or avoids, the brute fact remains that the fetus shifts and alters the very physical boundaries of the woman's self.

The women of the Good Birth Project agree, though vary widely in how they construe that pre-birth relationship. For Simone, it turns out, being inhabited felt good. "I loved pregnancy," she told us, "for the way it made me feel more . . . complete. The whole world was going on around you, but then there is this little thing moving inside of you, and it's just a moment in time that you share together. So it felt like me, but even better." For Christina, on the other hand, pregnant after years of infertility, *occupation* was more the point. "I pretty much just lay there. I'd had in vitro—there's something wrong with me. I'm not going to move around—I can't lose this baby."

The point is that, once we put pregnancy and how it's experienced into the picture, delivery seems more aptly described not as an arrival, but as a pulling apart and coming together, a sequential rending and re-forming of one of life's most intimate connections. If some people describe the process of bonding as "cementing" a woman and baby together, that depiction seems at best odd if you think about the fact that the two have just been held together for months on end by something much more robust, more thoroughgoing than cement.

So in our much-improved approach to bonding, we have perhaps forgotten to some extent the *rending* part of the equation—the fact that birth involves not just the grand occasion to connect with a new person, but the inevitable fact of physical separation from them. If emerging from the womb is, in the words of pediatrician and attachment parenting guru Bill Sears, a "harrowing experience" for babies, the presumption is that for women the experience is predominantly understood and experienced as a joyful union. Yet for some, it is feelings of separation—even *loss*—that mark the day or at least the first moments, and reasonably so.

The big lesson is that we just won't get it right if we don't consider that birth itself involves separation. "We come apart," writes Erica Jong, "that we may come together." For many women, birth makes us deal with the new fact of space between. It brings up that nagging truth that we really are, though for nine months accompanied, fundamentally alone. Perhaps this was the case for Simone, who during pregnancy felt "complete" but now with birth felt—not surprisingly to me—a loss, even though she had a baby girl in arms.

Or for Katha, who had gestated her baby for nine months, but now was dealing with the reality of nurses with needles and doctors with knives that had come between them. No wonder sitting with her baby felt painful—my sense is that there was more to it than the cesarean wound. With birth, they had been pulled apart, and the new space between them was filled with worry, with unthinkable possibilities that come with newborn heart surgery, with interventions well beyond her control, with the potential for a certain, almost unimaginable loss.

Brenda, who gave birth vaginally, but whose baby needed resuscitation because of a knot in the umbilical cord, told us that though she understood why her baby had to be tended in the nursery, it undid her. Birth felt distinctively like separation.

> What bothered me most was having to wait to see my baby again. Maybe an hour had passed, and I was like, "I really need to see my baby. I feel something is missing, like something has been disconnected. Obviously, it's my baby." I just felt like something was missing. I never realized that I would feel this huge connection of like, "If he's not in the room, I'm lost." Because he's been with me for nine months.

Karla reported a similar sensation when she reflected on the moments after the birth of her first of six children.

> I remember, with my first child very distinctly, crying with sadness. Sadness because this person's not inside of me anymore. Literally, it was such a separation anxiety. It was so horrible. I was like, "Wow, I'm really going to miss this person that was inside of me. What am I going to do now?"

I understand completely where Karla was coming from. This is where my head and heart took me during my pregnancies as well. I loved that feeling of being accompanied, all the time, and as splendid as it was to meet and gaze upon and smell that baby I'd gotten used to carrying, there was a certain loss in giving birth, in learning to share my boys with the rest of the world, in dealing with the fact that we were two, instead of one. In fact, sociologist Barbara Katz Rothman has offered provocatively that women "don't feel babies arrive, we feel them leave."

But this is only part of the truth. For some women, birth really does feel like just the beginning—and what happens in the delivery room feels very much like an arrival. It did for Karla in later births, in which she told us she felt "only gratitude. Gratitude and joy." This was also the case for Corey, who told us that she didn't feel particularly connected to her fetus during pregnancy; it was the moment of delivery when she felt her presence.

> When I was pregnant, it was really hard to think about something being in there, a human being being inside you. Even when we would do ultrasounds, it just looked weird. You're not really like, "That's my baby." So [the first moment I saw her] to me was the moment when I was like, "Oh my God, she's here."

Mother of four Eloise, who is also a close friend of mine, felt the same way. She told us:

> I think there are a lot of people who completely connect with their fetus. But for me, I don't talk to my babies when they are inside, put music on for them, or whatever people do. But I'm immediately connected to the baby at the birth. For me, the major part of the bonding is right at birth.

Whether giving birth feels to you more like separation, connection, or a mixture of the two, it seems to me that for many of us something more complicated than "bonding" is going on when we look upon the children we've just delivered. Simply denying that birth involves loss won't help us. There *is* something to be lost, and feeling that loss is normal; the shift in spaces shared between woman and baby is profound.

Kim has said (lovingly) of Eloise that "she goes through life on a surfboard—if it's below the surface, it doesn't exist." Of course, surfers will tell you that what's under the surface has everything to do with your ride and the way you make it to the shoreline. If the north-of-the-surfboard approach helps ease anxiety leading into delivery, denying the possibility of feeling a loss in birth can be a source of long-standing feelings of disappointment, buried sadness, and shame. We should remember instead that birth juxtaposes attachment and separation, and navigating *those* choppy waters well is ultimately key to getting to the good in birth.

No doubt one way to counterbalance that sense of loss is to get moms and babies together quickly after birth, just as we are doing—give them time and space to *re*connect in all the ways that we can and do post-birth. If that can happen and happen well, it's wonderful, and dozens of women told us how much they valued first moments, how absolutely central connecting quickly and deeply was to their sense that their birth was good. Finding our way (back) to our new babies is a big part of what the good birth is all about.

Ultimately, if connecting to baby is important to our sense that a birth is good, it's important to remember the conundrum it marks. Part of parenting is negotiating a certain sort of inevitable loss that comes with the growing love for our children. They are pulled from us, even as early as the moment a newborn is taken away for tests and cleaning; a baby is placed into to the arms of a loving friend; a child says good-bye on the first day of kindergarten; a young person falls in love. If it is true of birth, it is also true of parenthood: part of being a mother—and a father—is negotiating an inevitable tension between attachment and letting go.

Connecting to Loved Ones, Inside the Birthing Suite

The women of the Good Birth Project tell us that a good birth is one in which they feel connected to loved ones—intimate partners and close family in particular. But that can be more challenging than first meets the eye.

When we interviewed Corey before birth, it took her a while to tell us what was on her mind. She spent a lot of time saying what first-time moms often say—how she didn't want a C-section, how she hoped she wouldn't tear, how the most important thing to her was a healthy baby. But toward the end of our conversation, she disclosed her biggest fear, the "unknown factor," as she called it: her husband, Dan.

"I'm just glad it's not basketball season," she told us. Dan was an avid fan, and "worst-case scenario," she'd imagined, "was that he drops me off at the hospital, then goes to the game." She was half joking, of course. But as she went on, what became pretty clear was how birth felt to Corey like a test of their relationship, or more to the point, a threat to it. As she put it:

> It was very hard for me when I first got pregnant. I had a lot of concerns about how this would change our marriage . . . It's intimacy in a whole 'nother way. I worry about stretch marks and cellulite and never seeming attractive again to this person you're intimate with. And that is a really scary thing for me. I'm worried about the blood, about the loss of control you can have, of being that vulnerable, that way, to him.

Of being abandoned. We all are, to some extent. But for Corey, the prospect of giving birth brought those fears into sharp relief.

It's no wonder. If giving birth marks a major shift in the relationship between a woman and the child she carried for nine months, it also marks a major shift in relationships that have shaped her life for much longer, on the "outside," so to speak. And a good birth, many women tell us, is one in which they feel assured in the permanence of those pre-birth connections; a good birth is one in which we and our new babies are not alone—and won't be when we emerge on the other side as mothers.

How do we get that sense of connectedness? As Corey recognized in anticipation of delivery, it's not something most of us can orchestrate; it's another one of those elements in birth that are going to exceed control. You might have something in mind, and just have to let it go—like Eloise, who'd wished her husband, Cole, had shed a tear or two. "If I could have changed one thing," she reflected of her four births, "I would have had my husband be a little more emotional."

But there are things you can do—beginning, simply, with making sure the right person is present for delivery. For many women, that's their partner or spouse. And, of course, it's not just men anymore. Childbearing women—whatever their marital status—can in birth be accompanied by people other than the biological father of their child, especially if he is not the woman's partner, as is often the case with gay couples or women embracing single motherhood. Many women have more than one person they'd like to have in attendance, and these days the doors of delivery rooms have opened pretty widely. I've attended a good share of births in rooms crowded with friends and family. Even the most restrictive hospitals now allow at least two "visitors" of a mother's choosing if she delivers vaginally, and one by her side if she delivers by cesarean. Most freestanding birth centers leave the number of visitors up to parents. And if you are having a birth at home, of course, it's pretty much your call. You can invite the whole block, or close the shades and turn off the phone.

Part of why the evolution has been so important is that the alternative (isolation, aloneness) seems at best inhumane. But isolation is not just a thing of the past—and the women of the Good Birth Project who have given birth alone make no bones about the fact that feeling isolated or alone casts a pall on birth, regardless of the outcome. For instance, when her blood pressure skyrocketed in her first birth, Serena underwent a cesarean under general anesthesia. None of her family could be present for the birth, and going through that alone, Serena told us, "hurt"—clearly in more ways than one. When we asked her what makes for a good birth, she replied:

> I guess it's very important for you not to go through it alone. It's important for somebody to be there with you, besides the doctors and the nurses—somebody who should be there with you in the first place, someone who cares about you, from your family. It was very important for me for the second time, because I didn't have it the first time.

I suppose there are ways in which feeling alone in birth is inevitable. All of us who attend deliveries have witnessed (or experienced) the impulse some women have to flee. I remember during my residency one woman who was a push or two away from delivery telling us, "I've got to go, I've got to leave, I can't do this, leave me out of it"—and looking around frantically for the exit while we reminded her that her presence was essential, that she alone could give birth, that we were there to help, but we couldn't do it without her. Birth is in some ways inescapable—it is the woman alone who gestates, labors, and gives birth, whether or not she is surrounded by helping hands and empathic hearts.

Yet none of us wants to go through life events by ourselves—if we are scared, we want reassurance; if we are in awe, we want someone there to bear witness; if we feel vulnerable, we want someone there to shore us up. Birth is no exception. What's less obvious is what exactly these intimate others should do.

For some women, a loved one's presence is all they need, even if the other person doesn't say or do much of anything. Alex said having her husband there "does something for your peace of mind. That you're not in it alone—even though you're going through the pain alone, you know you can have someone that cares. You know what I mean?"

But if Corey's worries are any indication, the mere entry of intimates into the delivery room doesn't guarantee a good birth, and might even strain it if things don't go well. It's not just about having the right person there, but having them participate in a way that brings us closer, makes us feel helpfully supported and genuinely accompanied.

Like almost everything else in birth, there's no formula. If it's hard to predict what makes two people connect over a cup of coffee or on a seaside walk, connecting in birth brings heightened challenges. It depends on the relationship, what its strengths and chafe points are, what sorts of things bring you together, and how the two (or more) of you relate outside the birthing room. It is also shaped by the sort of birth you have, and what that birth demands or allows of a loved one and the space you share.

Nevertheless, there are lessons that run through births, good and bad, that can help facilitate connectedness in birth. For one, most of us want to feel like the person with whom we are about to parent is involved in birth in some meaningful way—we want our partners to *participate*.

For some women, that will mean engaging their husband or partner as a labor coach—a support person to help them breathe and cope with labor pain. Leslie took a Bradley class in preparation for her first delivery and really liked their approach. Bradley, or "husband-coached natural childbirth," is a method that involves partners through the process and brings them in to support women in anesthesia-free delivery. Leslie was hoping to deliver without pain medication and appreciated how Bradley engaged her husband in helping her meet that goal. Reflecting on her first birth, Leslie told us:

I don't think I could have done my first birth without my husband. He was more than just a labor coach. He was able to tell when I went into different stages of labor, he knew when to call, he knew when we needed to go. I literally did—like literally—physically lean on him during contractions, and he was very strong.

But not everybody wants their partner to take on that role. Wren, who wanted her husband there, hoped he would be able to cut the cord, but that was about it. She was most comfortable, she said, being able to depend on "good, supportive nurses" to coach her through the process.

I mean, my husband is wonderful, but he's not one of those "Go, honey, go! Go, honey, go!" kind of guys. Oh my God, I would die if he did that, you know? "Oh, shut the hell up!" I looked to the medical staff, because they know what's going on. I looked to them for my signals, for my support, for my "Am I okay?" kind of thing.

As different as their relationships (inside and outside the birthing suites) were, Leslie and Wren had remarkably similar reflections about what having their husband there—supporting them in a way that felt authentic—did for them. Both told us the experience brought them closer; both felt like having their husbands there changed something about how they related, changed how they were seen, and for the better. Leslie told us, "His level of respect for me just grew immensely—that I could do that. I don't want to toot my own horn, but he just couldn't stop talking about it for a few weeks." Similarly, Wren told us that after birth, "I looked at my husband and I could tell he was very proud of me. And that made me happy—that made me very happy."

A lesson for partners and loved ones here: If you are amazed or proud or moved in birth by what a childbearing woman does, let her know, tell her how you feel. It can mean the world to her.

What we found in listening to women is that there are countless ways to connect, and countless things to connect over, which range from the joyful to the terrifying. The key through the joys and uncertainties of birth is feeling genuinely accompanied; the challenge is figuring out how.

Sometimes a woman can seek out an insightful provider to lead the way. My sister-in-law Diane told me that one of the things she appreciated most about the midwife who attended the delivery of their first child, Jane, was the way in which she engaged my brother in the process. "He was scared out of his mind," Diane confided, "and he didn't know what to do. And I didn't know what to do for him." She went on to explain that their midwife, Kate, knew what both of them needed. She involved Mike throughout the course of Diane's pregnancy, and then with a grand gesture in birth, she took a step back from Diane as baby Jane was crowning, and allowed Mike to step in and catch his daughter. "It was the most emotional moment in either of our lives," Diane told to me. And when their Netflix offerings run out, one of their favorite things to do together is watch the video of Jane's birth. No doubt it is a tie that binds.

Now, I will tell you that this hands-on approach never appealed to me. I'm not bothered by the image of my brother in close proximity to my sister-in-law's vagina—that doesn't faze me in the least. And Kim and I both do love to look at the (still) images captured at each of our children's births. It's not that Kim wasn't scared; of course he was—being a doctor doesn't impart that sort of confidence (in fact, we have a better sense of what can go wrong). Indeed, there have been no days in our life together that I needed him more than the days our children were born.

But as willing as Kim was to do anything needed in the delivery room, and as utterly competent as he would be to make an incision or pop out a stuck shoulder if circumstances demanded, what was important to me was that he acted and felt like a husband and a dad, *not* a doctor, on the days our children were born. So I've always put him in charge of taking pictures, at least a lens away from the surgeon role he was used to playing in operating rooms. I saddled Kim with the camera because I just wanted him to be present as a partner, with his eyes on me and off the monitors, and as a dad, looking over the blue drape and seeing not a surgical field but the birth of our baby.

Could he have caught our boys? Most certainly. But a good birth for me, when it came to Kim, was his presence with me, on the north end of the blue drape, snapping precious photos of someone else pulling Grant, Paul, Charlie, and William from my body. The pictures, with each, have been brilliant—and so has Kim.

No single approach will work for every relationship. Some partners will be great coaches; others will find they need support themselves. For plenty of people, the sight of blood or a loved one in pain is unsettling and they end up propped in a corner with a cup of juice. That's okay. Brian, one of my closest friends in medical school, fainted during the first cesarean he witnessed (as a student, not a dad), and the nurses knew the drill so well that nobody in the room noticed what had happened except him and me. Though his nerves strengthened throughout his subsequent training (he's now a cardiologist), let's just say he remained "far from the business end" when his wife gave birth, ten years later.

For some women, hiring the right doula to act as a coach or advocate can free up intimates to connect with them and the baby in ways that feel authentic and meaningful to everyone. If you are giving birth, a doula might give your partner some pointers about how to support you, or might lift a burden of worry by explaining to you both what is happening, freeing your partner up to take part in what's happening and experience the event as momentous rather than confusing. The doula can provide physical assistance in labor, so your partner can focus on what you need emotionally. She can help your partner find the scrubs and the way to the operating room if you are headed there quickly for a cesarean; she can get your partner by your side and with presence of mind.

As beneficial as they can be for some, doulas aren't right for everyone. Some people want their partners to provide "labor support"—to be the coach, to attend to them, to be their advocate. Others just want to keep hands and hearts—however caring—to a minimum; extra hands can feel intrusive. For others, doulas have a particular time, place, and role—and a good one will have a sense of what is needed from her. Cara, a huge fan of what her doula did for her while she was in the hospital during her first birth, was convinced that the arrival in her home of a different doula in a subsequent birth made her labor stop—it disrupted the intimacy she and her husband had forged in her first hours of laboring together at home. The doula got the message, retreated, and allowed Cara and her husband to "get right back into it. We really had a rhythm—the two of us were like a machine."

There is no one "right" way to feel connected to a spouse or close family member. What's important, women tell us, is simply finding a way to connect—or stay feeling connected—in the process of birth. If you think a doula will help you feel that way, by all means consider hiring one. Some forward-thinking health programs will even offer them as a matter of course. If having another relative stranger in intimate space feels like a threat to such intimacy (as it might for introverts like me), it might not be the right thing for you.

Nor will a single approach work for every birth. Indeed, birth often defies our plans—but that need not leave us feeling alone. Women's stories indicate that there are many opportunities to connect that we cannot orchestrate. A good birth, then, requires a certain openness to the opportunities that emerge.

For instance, Leslie's third birth didn't leave any time for Rich to do his usual "coaching." Before she delivered, the two had flipped through the Bradley book, but were busy with their other two children and hoped husband-coached birth would be akin to riding a bike. But their lack of "preparation" didn't end up mattering, for other reasons entirely. When Leslie's water broke one afternoon at her sister's house, Rich's role was to drive the three of them at breakneck speed to the birth center, where Leslie delivered within five minutes of their arrival. But still, she explained:

> I felt like it was a bonding experience for all three of us. It went so fast and it was just this whirlwind and we all walked through it together. And it was just so joyous when it was over. That night I couldn't sleep very well, and I'd wake up and my sister would be awake, and Rich would be awake and we'd all have smiles on our face, and we relived what had just happened. It was just a really great time. We've never been closer.

Mara and her husband, Jake, discovered as much during the birth of their first child. They had attended Lamaze classes and together had crafted a role for Jake that involved "breathing techniques and the counting, and reminding me to focus—stuff he was sort of supposed to do." All that went by the wayside when she found herself headed to the operating room for an emergency cesarean. No doubt, having Jake by her side was reassuring. But for Mara, there was more—a deeper sense of connectedness that was forged in the process. As she put it:

> When things went downhill, I just remember, I had the breathing mask over me and he was like right up in my face, holding my hand, saying, "It's going to be okay, it's going to be okay." I remember he was crying, and I've never seen him cry before. It was just, I don't know, one of those life moments.

Perhaps even more surprising to her, Jake's being in the operating room with her allowed her to see things through him she couldn't see for herself, to capture a vantage point that would have been lost but for his presence.

> I couldn't see the birth and I had wanted to see it, so [Jake] stood up and took a picture when Jacob was coming out. He got these horribly gory, bloody pictures that I love. But even better, he was so excited. I could see what was happening sort of reflected in his face—he was sitting back behind me. Just to see him react and be so loving toward our baby right away, it was just wonderful.

We heard this time and again from the women of the Good Birth Project, whatever their delivery mode, and whatever their husband or partner's particular role—coach or cord cutter, photographer or baby catcher. They relished their partner's excitement about the birth, they loved "seeing" birth through the eyes of someone similarly moved by it, they loved the fact that being so moved was something they shared. First-time mom Halle, who had a quick vaginal birth in the hospital, told us of her husband, Drew:

> He was wonderful. He was really more excited, I think, than I was. He was seeing it from a different perspective . . . I was getting excited from his excitement, looking at him watch her head pop out. And he's like, "Oh, she has hair and I think I see her!" And so it was really wonderful having him there.

And it wasn't just husbands or intimate partners. Mother of four Josie told us that one of the things she loves about one video taken of her giving birth is that you can hear, ever so softly, the videographer—her sister—weeping as her niece's head emerged.

But there were other things—beyond coaching, beyond shared experience, that made the presence of intimate others important. Lindsey, for instance, told us that her husband's presence gave her a sense of "stability"—that there was someone there who knew her, who had her back.

> That was nice, having him there. He provided a sense of stability . . . Knowing I had someone to support me when I needed it was great. Knowing I had someone who was going to advocate totally for me and the baby was good. Knowing that he would understand whatever they were talking about was a relief. It kind of helped me realize that, if there were truly a big emergency, he could have made the decisions that needed to be made, and I wouldn't have to worry about that.

And mother of six Karla told us that her husband's presence at her last birth—which was also her first cesarean—was more important to her than in any of the births that preceded it, even though she ended up being under general anesthesia for its entirety. She told us:

> Knowing that he was there was so important. It was so important. Him being there, just saying, "It's going to be okay." Literally thinking in my mind, "If I don't make it—but I know I will, because he's here." When I closed my eyes and went to sleep, remembering him and his face and our experience were just the most memorable things about that occasion.

Finally, it's important to remember that some intimacies are best maintained through a loved one's absence—rather than their presence. This was rarely if ever the case with partners or spouses, but I can imagine there are exceptions. A good share of women who were close to their mothers (and fathers) maintained that it was critical to them that they *not* be in the room—that being seen in pain, exposed, by parents (or children) would be disruptive to relationships they held dear. "My parents stood outside the room until the head came out, and then they came in," said Wren. "That's how I wanted it to be."

In fact, for her second birth, Wren's parents didn't quite make it to the hospital, which unexpectedly cleared the way for other intimacies. "So it was just my husband and I, so it was really kind of special and neat. We got to spend those first moments, just the three of us, so that was kind of cool."

No doubt, birth changes close relationships. But Corey discovered that, while she was right about birth changing things, it can also provide occasion and experience that makes a relationship better. In fact, she told us in her postpartum interview that her birth—her good birth—was so very good because of that. "Everything," she told us, "turned out totally opposite, and so wonderful." She explains:

> One of my fears was about my husband being there, and how it would change our relationship. Well, it did. It brought us closer than ever. He held my leg and watched her head crown. I'm crying now, but he was crying. It was incredible. It just made me feel like I could do it, and that I wasn't alone. That's probably the biggest thing, that I wasn't alone.

These days, if Kim and I hug while I have Will on my hip, the sentiment between the two is all too clear: Will's palm presses against Kim's chest, and Kim channels good-naturedly, "Back off, Dad." Or my brother's familiar exchange with my five-year-old nephew when he wraps himself around my sister-in-law: "Get your own wife, buddy," to which Laird replies, "Get your own mom." There is always room in our heart, but sometimes things can feel a little crowded; there is always a way to hold on, but birth makes us want to make sure we can.

Connectedness to Health Care Professionals

I'll admit, I'm friends—good friends—with some of the women who were once my patients. Making friends with patients is one of those things in medicine that feels and is often considered taboo. There are obvious reasons for this when romance is involved, but even when it's not, cautions are raised about whether the imbalance of power and knowledge between doctors and patients makes their friendship impossible. I've always done my best to level the field on both counts, and have come to the conclusion that I've learned much more from the women I've cared for than they ever could have learned from me. I'm not sure whether that justifies my crossing fine lines, but it does make me feel that the eschewing of friendship where it's arisen would be harder still to justify.

Emotions can overwhelm when it comes to birth, and just to function we doctors find ways to stiffen our upper lip—something I came to appreciate in the midst of the first birth I witnessed in medical school, during a pediatrics rotation. I was a student in the neonatal intensive care unit, and the pediatrics team was called to a woman's birth in which meconium (dark green staining of amniotic fluid) had appeared, indicating that the baby was stressed in labor. The team's job was to ensure that the child didn't inhale the offending fluid with its first breath; my job as the quivering med student was to transport the baby from the birthing table to the nearby pediatricians. I was told to stand at the foot of the bed and hold my arms out straight in front of me, upon which a green cloth and (moments later) the slippery newborn were placed. But in the moments I saw the baby's head emerge and felt its weight in my arms, my eyes filled up with tears and I could hardly see where to walk. "This," I thought, "is not going to work. I've got to toughen up."

Of course, I wasn't connected in any way to the woman giving birth—I didn't even know her name. But as I started to get to know my patients, negotiating—and, perhaps more to the point, containing the emotions that birth evokes—seemed critical to professional comportment, and I did my best for a while, figuring out at least how to contain tears.

I discovered, however, that it's not so black-and-white. If the detached but competent physician is accepted as the norm in some areas of medicine, patients tell us that birth is a place in which closer connections are key. As mother of two Liz put it, "There's a major difference in your relationship with your doctor between having some sort of illness and having this major life experience. It's kind of like an intimate thing."

I'm not sure I think that birth is as exceptional as Liz describes—medicine is full of intimacies. In surgery, we dip our hands into patients' bodies; in diagnosing and treating medical illness, no doubt we touch bodies and lives and become a part of them. Nevertheless, birth is widely accepted as an intimate experience, both for its physical particularities and its place in our lives.

To the extent that doctors resist intimacy, their resistance has some powerful detractors. My colleague Jodi Halpern, a philosopher and psychiatrist, has spent much of her professional life arguing that empathy in the setting of health care is critical to getting (and giving) good and humane care. Doctors, she argues, need two things: genuine curiosity about how their patient is feeling and emotional connection with them.

The women of the Good Birth Project seem to agree. They tell us that part of having a good birth is feeling emotionally connected to health care providers—to people in attendance other than partners, family, or close friends. Of course, we want and need the professionals who attend our births to be present and competent and keep us safe through the process, to practice obstetrics or midwifery responsibly and respect our wishes. But many women say that what made their birth good was how intimate it felt—in part because of how deeply connected they felt to the people whose job it was to catch their baby or wipe their brow.

For instance, Simone repeatedly described her second birth as "romantic." Part of what made it feel that way was the absence of the chaos that had characterized her first birth—no emergencies, no pain (she had an epidural), no forceps—just a gentle if anesthetized birth. But part of what made it feel romantic was how she felt about who was there. She explains:

> It was the most romantic delivery on the face of the earth. It was just me, the doctor, my husband. I went into labor, had the epidural, could have stayed in labor four days—I couldn't care. The doctor I knew stayed late for the delivery . . . It was small, it was

intimate, and it was like a family member delivering me, and it was really special . . . We were all kind of laughing, I was relaxed, I felt fabulous.

If Simone's experience sounds exceptional, it has seemed to me that this sort of intimacy is not so hard for midwives; it is perhaps even the norm. In fact, for many midwives I've spoken to, cultivating intimacy appears to be part and parcel of their approach to maternity care. Many pride themselves on the degree to which they connect with patients—before, during, and after birth. Patients are friends, friends are patients, and birth brings them together. Midwives' appointments tend to be longer; understanding patients' lives in their messiness and depth seems to be critical to good midwifery. One of the midwives we interviewed made me want to have my baby at her birth center (despite the medical imprudence of doing so after three cesareans), just so I could connect with her, so I could feel what it was like to have her take care of me. From what I understand, she has had this effect on many if not most of the women with whom she's crossed paths. She explained her approach:

> We sit down in our room together [and I tell my patient] that we're going to be a team, we're going to be partners. I need to know about your partner, what his or her expectations are, I want to meet your mother, I want to meet your grandmother. If you want your kids there, I want to meet them too. We can really talk and look at the best possible birth that we're going to work together to get, and that's all I can give people.

And then, wiping her tears aside, she told us, "I cry at people's births all the time. When babies are born and Daddy cries, oh, I'm a goner. I'm a birth junkie—I don't know. I just love it." So much for my stiff upper lip.

Another midwife, Kitty Ernst, projects something similar. When Emily, my research colleague in the Good Birth Project, and I visited Kitty at the midwifery school she directs in Kentucky, within moments of greeting, pregnant Emily spontaneously and wordlessly decided to lift her sweater so that Kitty could lay hands on her belly. It was a moment I'll always remember, especially given that Emily and I often exchanged stories and disdain about how people feel like bellies are in the public domain, and that I'd known Emily to otherwise recoil at many an outstretched hand. There was just something about Kitty, though, that made Emily want to connect with her.

Mandy talked about the midwives who attended her second birth at home, which she said was exceptionally good.

> I had people there who I love and who love me and who were also very competent and capable. I mean, any of those midwives, except one, could have been my mother, but better. Because I love my mother and she's local, but she could never have been like that for me, in labor.

But I am reluctant to make too much of the way midwives and doctors are characterized respectively. For one, there are exceptions—plenty of them, like midwives who fail to connect. Mandy had one of those in her first birth—she felt that she was "neglected," that "nobody was really doing anything for me," and, perhaps most tellingly, that in retrospect, "maybe I didn't trust my first midwife so much." And women tell us that there are in fact doctors who do connect brilliantly—Simone, for one, certainly would say that. Some people say the former are aberrations, and the latter are "midwives in disguise." I suppose that is one way to think about it.

Yet there is a bigger problem with reifying that distinction between midwives and doctors: midwives are usually associated with low-risk births, but women with complicated births need to feel connected too—in fact, I might argue that they need it *more*. Women need and deserve to feel connected whether they've spent hours with a midwife planning an out-of-hospital birth, or less time meeting the dozen doctors that make up a group hospital practice. Consider in particular women who need care from a doctor because birth presents dangers for them or their babies—like Katha, whose baby was born with a heart defect; or Jill, who mid-pregnancy went into liver failure and needed a cesarean to save her life and that of her baby. You might say that if anyone needed to feel cared for and connected, it was these two women, though their births were far from "natural." If competency in obstetric medicine was necessary, it was far from sufficient to a good birth.

Jill—who had about as complicated and "medical" a birth as one could imagine—did feel connected. Her doctor was one of the few high-risk obstetricians in this country who is in fact a "midwife in disguise"—she had actually practiced midwifery for fifteen years before training in maternal-fetal medicine. But if Jill was fortunate to land in hands that were both caring and competent, I can vouch for the fact that her doctor is not an aberration, that a good many of my colleagues know how to connect as well. Jill had been transferred by ambulance to a major medical center and had never met any of the people who'd be doing her cesarean in the moments after her arrival. But she told us, "I had faith in the hospital, in the doctors, right away." She explained:

> My doctor there was very serious, gave me her full attention.
> Everybody was very caring, showing empathy. I felt like they
> saw me as a person and were attentive to my needs. Everyone
> was just very caring—it gave me a calmness about it.

This is all to say that birth is unpredictable and intimacies will need at times to be forged in short order; women shouldn't have to rely exclusively on long-standing relationships with trusted midwives or the rare "midwife in disguise." The person who performs the emergent cesarean incision, who dips the hand in the body, who places needed forceps, is in intimate space. If some need reminding, many of us know it. Forging connectedness is as important for the physician performing decidedly "medical" procedures as it is for the midwife whose job description has traditionally demanded that relationship.

While in conducting the Good Birth Project we heard about the importance of connecting to providers across all kinds of women and all kinds of births, it turned out to be especially important for women without a close companion with them in labor, and their numbers are not insignificant. More and more women are deciding to have children on their own—I know several (one a very good friend) who amid the din of the biological clock decided to get pregnant with sperm purchased on the Internet. Another friend was separated from her husband weeks after she found out she was pregnant. Women will labor while partners are overseas or just scrambling, sometimes unsuccessfully, to meet them in the hospital.

Natasha went into labor two months early with her first baby, and her husband was out of town on a business trip. A neighbor brought her to the hospital, where she delivered within a few hours. "I was scared," she told us, "because it was my first child, and his dad wasn't going to be there. That's what made me disappointed—he wasn't there for the birth." But she was grateful for the way the nursing staff stepped in.

> None of my family or anybody was there with me. It was just nurses. And they were around me the whole time. So that was a big part of what made it okay—the emotional support. You know, they helped me. Even though I was crying and asking for my husband, they told me, "It's okay, this baby's coming if he's here or not." They would tell me, "We're here. *Right now, we're your family.*"

Ming also felt alone in labor, and looked to (and felt grateful for) nurses who made extra efforts to make her feel more accompanied. Ming, who had grown up in China, was working in a research laboratory in the United States and had married an American who turned out to be less than supportive during and after birth. "I don't know if it's his being American," she reflected, "but he was like a boy. He didn't know how much pain I was in—he didn't understand how hard it was. When I asked him to pass me water, he would complain." But the nurses stepped in, and they were a big part of what made the experience good. Like Natasha's nurses, Ming referred to them as "family."

> There was a lady I remember—she's from the Philippines. I think she was one of the best nurses I ever had. She was very genuine, always smiled . . . I just feel like she's very close to me, *just like part of your family.* Not just someone professional, like, "Oh, okay, I'm working here." I mean, that kind of relationship is different. The feeling that I have is like they really care about you.

If critical for Ming and Natasha, this more intimate feeling of assistance was important to women even when they had supportive partners or family at the ready. The challenge was how to assure those connections to providers at those crucial crossroads. Again, it's hard to orchestrate. For instance, nobody gets to choose their nurses. It's luck of the draw, leading to the conclusion that Natasha and Ming both lucked out. Thank goodness their nurses stepped in—otherwise they'd really have been alone, and their births might have been more like the one that brought my friend Ben to tears.

And as much as we wish it were otherwise, it's getting harder to choose your doctor or midwife. Most practice in groups, so even if you find a kindred spirit in a health care provider, there's no guarantee she'll be there at the birth; it might just be one of her partners. One midwife who runs a popular practice (and who is known if pressed to pull multiple nights in a row) told me that she has to assure her patients that she never hires a midwife she wouldn't herself welcome into her own delivery. But if the women she hires are trustworthy and competent, there's no guarantee any two people will connect on a personal level, especially when stakes are high.

But how can a woman make certain she feels connected—enough—to the people caring for her? Again, this can be a way that a doula may come in handy. If you hire one before birth, you can make sure you like her, and may be able to pay for the assurance she'll be there at your birth. But they are not right for everyone or might not be available or affordable. And as we saw in Chapter 3, when doulas are hired to "run interference," they can reinforce distance between women and doctors that many of us find detrimental to the good birth.

No doubt we health care providers—doctors, midwives, nurses—need to remember how important it is to make our patients feel supported, accompanied, and we need to make that a priority in how we care for women giving birth. Birth is no time to keep our distance.

But if you are heading toward birth, what else can you do? Begin by listening to yourself. Pay attention to how you feel about the doctor or midwife who is most likely to be at your delivery. Do you feel like you relate to them? Do they inspire confidence? Do they make you want to lift up your sweater like Emily did? Do you want them at this major life event? Do they feel anything to you like family (and if so, is that a good thing)? Of the midwife who attended her second delivery, Mandy told us, "When she walked in the door, I was like, *aah*. That feeling came over me, like now I know things are going to be okay."

Also, be as open as you can to forging new connections in the process of birth. You might zero in on a favorite doctor or midwife before delivery, but the way most practices are structured these days, there is a reasonable chance he or she won't be the person attending your birth. But not getting the attendant you want is not the end of the world. Several women of the Good Birth Project were surprised at what birth brought out in people who attended their births—even midwives or doctors who weren't, in clinic visits, their "favorite." Many of us providers still are riding upon some bit of wonder when we attend births, and it can emerge during delivery in surprising ways.

Finally, most of the time there will be more than one attendant in the room who can give you the connection you may need in birth. If it feels like it is not forthcoming from the surgeon at work on your belly or the midwife between your legs, remember that there are other people who are there to support you. Ming and Natasha connected with their nurses; I was, myself, surprised at how connected I felt to the anesthesiologists who placed my epidurals. I remember every one, and am (nearly) as grateful for the ways they seemed to care about me and my birth as I was for their accuracy with regard to my spinal cord. Like so many of life's attachments, connectedness cannot be planned or forced, but a little faith and openness can go a long way.

Connections Outside the Birthing Suite

Okay, my mom did this, my grandmother did this, the Pilgrims did this. Granted, we've had varying success with morbidity and mortality, but it's fascinating to think that that's what makes us the same.

—COLBY, OBSTETRICIAN

Birth is not just concerned with relationships inside the birthing room— there are relationships outside that also shape birth, and are shaped by birth. So a good birth, women tell us, is one that allows us to maintain our connectedness to certain other people—people who, if not immediately involved in our births, are a part of our lives. And we want them to stay that way.

That connectedness was the thing that ultimately determined where my colleague Etta gave birth. Etta is fiercely independent, as evidenced by her decision to conceive at thirty-nine with sperm she ordered on the Internet. A practicing obstetrician and professor at a major U.S. medical school, she actually preferred to give birth at home. She knew what hospital birth entailed and wanted something different. She liked the privacy that home birth offered, had a midwife she knew well and trusted, and had close friends who could support her. A breathtaking intellect, she had slashed through the framing and rhetoric that complicates birth debates and felt utterly comfortable that home birth was safe for her.

But Etta knew that her professional colleagues didn't agree and would never understand her choice. She told me, "I don't think I could face my partners if I delivered at home." So she labored in her cozy townhome until she was nine centimeters dilated and then went to the hospital, where she pushed Lily into the hastily gloved hands of her colleague. Sure, it was a compromise, but it was the best way, Etta concluded, to have the experience she wanted without having to deal with a professional-identity-shaping aftermath.

Etta's decision about that last-minute transfer—given how independent she is, intellectually and otherwise—has always struck me as remarkable. She writes papers that turn heads and spark fury among colleagues; she raises questions on sensitive topics that lead many of us to respect her not just for her hard and careful work but also for her bravery. And yet it was in birth (her *own* birth, no less) that she felt she needed to compromise to maintain her professional integrity.

Perhaps it reflects how deeply entrenched we are in the birth wars, how dangerous it feels to pull away from the usual ways of thinking and operating. All the more reason, it strikes me, to support those we care for and about in their efforts to do so. All the more reason to reorient around a new and authentic conception of the good birth.

Like it or not, how we give birth shapes how people perceive us, and thus how we relate to them. For many women, a good birth is a birth that works with who we are and how others see us. Perhaps more to the point, a good birth is one that allows us to stay connected to the people we loved, depended on, or just worked with before we delivered.

Sometimes, of course, that urge to stay connected can feel constraining. I don't know if Etta felt constrained by her compromise, but she's talked about it enough to make me think she did. She shouldn't have had to compromise. That we are judged, so profoundly, for our choices in birth is something that I hope is changing, and that I'd like to help change. That women will—and do—change their decisions at birth because people they love don't understand is part of what's wrong with how we talk about birth these days, an untoward and damaging consequence of the birth wars. Indeed, several of the women of the Good Birth Project told us that they thought there were "plenty of options" for women these days. The problem, though, was others' judgment, and the potential for blame. Simone put it this way:

> I think it can be hard for [moms]. They are trying to make this decision. They have friends that have delivered in a pool, or in a major medical center, or above a yoga studio. Pregnancy was just the hardest time for me in terms of being confident with myself and the decisions I wanted to make about where and how to deliver.

Mom of two Laurie told us that when she was pregnant with her first, all her girlfriends were into home birth—but she knew it wasn't for her. "I had no need for that," she told us. "I wanted drugs, I wanted an epidural, but I didn't know how I could do that and save face with my friends." In her third trimester, she and her husband unexpectedly moved to North Carolina. She found an OB practice, delivered with an epidural at a community hospital, and never looked back. Though she did admit she was glad that weight, length, and birth date were all that were required on the usual birth announcement. "It wasn't like I had to advertise that Dillon was born—gasp—in a hospital."

I will say, though, that there is nothing like having a baby or two to broaden a person's view about what birthing in one way or another means about a person. As I argued in Chapter 1, giving birth teaches us things about what we can control and what we can't. Worries about judgment are not unfounded, but I'd suggest it's reasonable to assume that birth imparts a wisdom and humility. Most of the women I've taken care of, and those with whom I work, jog, stand in line to pick up children at school—whose hearts and minds, and bodies, have been stretched and shifted by birth—will not be so quick to judge, having ridden birth's unpredictable wave.

My friend Jackie and I agree that yoga classes—if good for the gestating body—are fertile ground for judgment. This is particularly true when they are full of first-time moms who've been led to believe that if they take care of themselves (do yoga, eat quinoa), then they'll have just the sort of birth they planned—the forest bower version I mentioned in the Introduction. Jackie recalled feeling judged by one expectant mom who shared with the class her "devastation" at needing a cesarean for her breech baby. "I felt alienated. I felt the judgment just seeping out of her toward those of us who'd had cesareans, or those of us who didn't care quite as much about the natural birth process as she did." But, Jackie told me, post-birth they became friends, both wiser for having been through the process of birth and weathered its twists and turns, both humbled by the challenges of parenting, both forgiving of other women's choices. "That judgment," Jackie reflected, "if it was there at all, was minimized by all that we share in common. I don't feel judged by her, nor do I judge her." Finding our way around judgment can be tricky business, though, and I'll get to that in Chapter 5.

Birth can strain connectedness with other family members too. Many women wonder, when they are having their second child, how there really could be room in their heart for two when one seemed to fill it up so completely. Like Alex, who said:

> I had a little more anxiety with the second one. I think, being that I had an older child, I was worried about their feelings and how are they going to take to this new baby . . . I just had a little bit more stress on me the second time around, just because I was worried so much about my older son's feelings.

Most of us would tell Alex that hearts do stretch somehow, that there will be room even if life on the outside gets chaotic—that siblings for the most part are gifts to the children we have, if not at first, then eventually. And perhaps most to the point, that if having a second baby changes the way we see our first, few would say it disconnects. But birth can make you wonder, and assurance that those bonds are secure makes the process that much better. For some, all that takes is having someone around who can be with an older sibling and introduce the two at an opportune time. For others, it will mean having the child in attendance when their brother or sister enters the world. It also will shape decisions about how to deliver. For instance, Colleen had chosen a cesarean for her first birth, but was considering a VBAC for her second child. She explained:

> I knew I had a three-and-a-half-year-old at home and I was like, "What if I can't pick her up and she won't understand?" I think a large part of my decision was having the older child at home and thinking, "If I do a C-section . . . not only does she have to adjust to a baby, she has to adjust to 'Mom can't pick you up right now,'" and so that was the anxiety I had about having another C-section.

Other times, the urge to stay connected can just feel hard, as it did for Lucy, leading into her first birth. Her mom had recently been diagnosed with lymphoma and was too sick to visit—she had to be home in bed in another state the day that Lucy went into labor. Needless to say, it felt like a big loss going into birth. She'd wanted her mom there, she'd wanted to share it with her, and she wanted her to feel invited. But then, the unexpected happened.

Lucy had turned off her cell phone during labor; she didn't want everyone she knew checking in. Late in the day, her husband, Jake, made a trip to the cafeteria to get a bite of supper, and within minutes of his departure, she felt the urge to push. So she turned on the phone and called Jake to tell him to hurry back. The phone sat quietly at her bedside for the two hours it took to push her baby out. A minute after her daughter's birth, it rang.

> We looked at the screen—it was Mom. And I said to my husband, "Oh, pick up." So he picks up and she started to apologize, "I'm sorry, I didn't want to bother you. I'm just sitting on pins and needles." And then she heard [my daughter] cry. So, yeah, I guess she was sort of there. That was the part that was surprising to me. Because my mom said afterward, "Oh, and then I heard your voice and I knew you were okay."

Lucy got to share her birth with her mom, in a way she didn't orchestrate—couldn't have orchestrated. And yet that unexpected shared moment, she told us, was what made her good birth good. And that it mattered to her mother that she was okay brought the connections in her life into sharp relief: with the call came the recognition that she was a daughter and a mother at the same time.

Many women tell us that birth is a way that they can, and do, connect: to their moms, to other women, to humanity. Several told us they felt, having given birth, like they were finally "part of the club"—and that nothing but going through it opened that door. Others told us that pregnancy itself made them feel connected to other women, and that felt reassuring as they anticipated the prospect of pushing a fully formed baby out of their body. As seasoned midwife Donna puts it, "Hey, I did it, my daughter did it, my mother did it—you know women have been doing it from the beginning of time . . . Otherwise there wouldn't be the human race there is today." Hers was an assurance quoted time and again by the women we interviewed, whatever their birth mode. Birth connects us in certain ways to others, and that connectedness can help many of us through delivery, and reassure us when we emerge on the other side.

———

I feel the world has changed because of my baby. Before, I was always afraid of death. But now I feel, even if I die, I have someone.

—MING

"Not again, Mom, he's *fine*," my oldest son, Grant, would tell me, as I pulled over to the side of the road.

In his first months on the planet, Will hated being in the car—I mean, hated. And this is a problem when you have three other children who need to be shuttled back and forth every day to school, sports, piano, friends' houses.

In the first days of Will's protests, I'd stop the car—multiple times—just to make sure that his finger wasn't pinched in the restraints, or some sharp object was not breaking his skin (neither was ever the case). When he stopped howling, I'd stop again to check to be sure that he was still breathing (he always was). Although Grant, the first child, characteristically assumed the role of protector, our car trips were more punctuated than even he thought necessary to assure the health of all.

You'd think a mother of four would have thicker skin, but I just didn't. Will's cry sounded so mournful. It tugged at me, brought me back to the first days of his life, when he was "whisked away" to the intensive care unit. As he cried and I drove, I would imagine what those first days must have been like for him—alone in a bassinet, people sticking him with needles, a light in his face—and imagined him wondering (if babies wonder), Is this life? Is this how it is? Maybe, I thought, the car seat brought that back for him, a deep loneliness. Or maybe it brought loneliness back for me.

Loneliness is something everyone struggles against at some point, and we all have our ways of resisting it. For some people, the salve is good literature. "The deepest purpose of reading and writing fiction," offered writer Garth Risk Hallberg in an essay for the *New York Times*, "is to sustain a sense of connectedness, to resist existential loneliness."

For me it has been birth more than books, though I suppose that overflowing bookcases and toy boxes in our house betray a deep love and need for both on my part. In birth I've physically felt a consciousness independent of my own—this new negotiation between me and not me, knowing that now there is something, someone I'd willingly die for, this re-forming of myself in relation to another. In many ways, Will and his brothers are a buffer against an existential loneliness I've fought against all my life.

And I suppose that is why, despite Grant's reassurances, despite the illogic, I kept pulling over, until Will finally found comfort in his fuzzy gray car seat, and I again could feel assured that neither of us felt, for the moment at least, alone.

If other moms pull over, I hope they'll at least avoid that foray into loneliness that the events of Will's birth engendered. Another reason, perhaps, that we need to do our best to get it right at the beginning.

But I hope this chapter has made clear that birth doesn't have to occur a certain way, that there isn't a script for first moments, for intimate partners, for the maternity care providers that we hope will accompany us as we give birth. Rather, there are as many kinds of first moments as there are mothers and children. And there are just as many ways to feel connected to others besides the baby, to feel assured that we are not alone as we become parents. The key, I've come to believe, is holding fast to moments that are yours, rather than mourning them because they didn't live up to a particular ideal. Not stepping over photos, but picking them up as soon as we realize they have fallen to the ground.

five

Respect

It's not the end of the world if you have a cesarean. Most women are just fine and they still consider [their birth] a beautiful experience . . . You have to have given them the chance, you have to respect the woman, the process, the baby. If she knows that everyone's been respected and everyone's done the best they could, that makes a big difference psychologically for the woman and how she experiences birth.

—ANNA, MIDWIFE

At last, with the birth of each daughter, Michael and I experience a certainty of apprehension, a sensation so profound that I feel foggy brained attempting to describe how, in the first moment after birth, the actual being of a new person appears.

—LOUISE ERDRICH

As I've mentioned, Kim is a surgeon, comfortable in an operating room and appreciative of what modern medicine can do for the birth process. Yet he often recalls with chagrin how the celebratory mood in the labor room changed when it became clear that I'd need a cesarean to deliver our first child, Grant.

I should explain that Kim did a surgical residency a couple of decades ago, at a time when "giants walked the halls" at Duke and training in surgery was understood and embraced as nothing short of harrowing. Most of his six years of training were spent doing thirty-six hours on, twelve hours off—hardly enough time to sleep and eat, much less regain a sense of humanity. Needless to say, he knows as well as anyone about how training in medicine can make a person retreat and put on a steely exterior, and is willing to forgive all measure of failures in that regard. But when it came to our first baby's birth, the failures had an enduring sting.

We loved a good part of the day. Of course, the morning had its frustrations—Kim had retreated at first to the operating room to take care of his patient with breast cancer. But by midday, he had put down his scalpel, found his way to me, and perhaps pressed some of his own uncertainties aside. I labored in a well-appointed labor, delivery, recovery, and postpartum (LDRP) room, more refined—and yes, homey—than the yet-to-be-updated historic house we'd recently purchased. I worked through contractions for a while, then got an epidural and settled into what I'd call joyful anticipation. Kim and I were having a baby. It was, no doubt, something to celebrate.

With evening upon us, my cervix was nearly fully dilated but Grant's head remained well above what we call the "pelvic brim"—bony prominences that doctors and midwives use as a reference point to describe how far a baby's head has descended into the birth canal. We knew he was a big baby; with his head nearly out of reach, a cesarean seemed prudent, perhaps inevitable, so with some prodding I agreed to it.

And with that, everyone went into surgery mode. Celebration was replaced by the familiar seriousness of an operating theater; in the midst of the uncomplicated surgery, congratulations were replaced by apologies. After a couple of hours in the recovery room, I was wheeled not to the new and conspicuously homelike LDRP room in which I'd labored all day, but to a small room in the next hallway over, alongside women who'd had not only cesareans, but others who'd had miscarriages and hysterectomies.

In the course of Grant's birth, there was good attention to one specific form of respect—what medical ethicists call *respect for autonomy*. People made sure I understood the procedure, agreed to it, and gave my consent for cesarean. But the way things went, I could just as well have been having an appendectomy. Something, a different sort of respect, it struck me (and Kim), was missing. What we didn't experience was respect for birth, for *our* birth.

As it turns out, it didn't have to be this way, and by the fourth time around—when I gave birth, again by cesarean, to William—I found my way to it, that missing piece. I found respect in and for birth. And when I thanked one of the obstetricians who did my fourth cesarean, she replied more than once, "It's a real honor to be here, Annie." I never got tired of hearing that.

There is a widespread assumption that if you give birth in a hospital—and especially if you give birth by cesarean—that birth will become a medical event, narrowly construed. Partly to blame is the fact that most things that occur in hospitals don't fit into the same—if you will—*sacrosanct* category of birth. And so when doctors, nurses—even midwives—shift into hospital mode, things like respect for birth can get lost.

This shift of gaze and attitude certainly could explain why resistance to "medicalizing" birth—treating birth as a medical event—has taken such hold. Many of the women we interviewed asserted that "pregnancy is not an illness." And diverse literatures and perspectives on the topic of birth hold that birth is "normal" and "non-pathological." True enough. But for a long time, this view, mobilized often in critiques of obstetrics and its approach to birth, confused me. If one in five apparently normal pregnancies require medical intervention to prevent harm to a woman or her baby, how could it be that when it comes to birth, medicalization is so inappropriate?

Part of the answer lies in what we in medicine tend to do when we don our white coats, what Kim and I saw in those who attended Grant's birth. Too often, we shove meaning to the side and make elimination of pathology our singular goal, even when that possibility is remote. With this orientation, the appropriately medical aspects of birth can eclipse everything else, and birth gets stuck in the category of a medical event.

Treating something as a medical event doesn't have to mean that the people involved are treated less than humanely. There are growing efforts to emphasize this—like the headline-grabbing $42 million gift to the University of Chicago for an institute to teach medical students better bedside manner. Still, when it comes to surgeons, affronts at the bedside are widely viewed as tolerable as long as technical skill is in place.

Not so in birth. Lack of bedside manner is much harder to overlook during this experience. Women want their doctors and midwives not just to be kind and compassionate, but also to see birth as extraordinary, celebrated, uncanny, supremely memorable. They want them to respect it. It is in this way—and in several others I'll describe in this chapter—that respect is key to a good birth. It was that missing piece from Grant's delivery—the piece I found when giving birth to Will.

What We Really Mean When We Talk About Respect

Even before I started the Good Birth Project, I understood that respect was critical to a good birth. The births I'd attended during residency where it appeared to be lacking had gotten under my skin and contributed to my affinity for midwives and their mantras—which almost always invoke the importance of respectful treatment and personal attention to the woman giving birth.

Respect has been emphasized in medicine as well, particularly as it relates to a doctor's duty to respect the informed preferences of patients—to respect their autonomy. Respect in this sense is the basis for informed consent, the requirement that doctors inform their patients about the options for care, relevant risks, benefits, and alternatives, and refrain from doing things that their patients refuse. Indeed, this is the type of respect I was absolutely afforded during my delivery with Grant.

But respect for autonomy—if important—doesn't capture fully what the women of the Good Birth Project say about respect when talking about a good birth. What comes through their stories is a conception of respect that is rich and multifaceted, directed toward not only the woman but also her new baby and toward birth itself as a major life event imbued with bodily and existential meaning.

Furthermore, respect as we usually think about it in medicine doesn't get at something else that is deeply at issue in birth: dignity. I think of dignity (from the Latin *dignitas*, or "worthiness") and respect as close companions. Dignity, as I understand it, is something about a person or an event that confers a sense of worthiness of due regard, that demands our respect. Sometimes dignity calls for respect on the part of others; other times it is related to the degree that we respect ourselves. As many have noted to be true about the other bookend of life, there is something about birth that makes women tighten their grip on dignity and, in certain circumstances, mourn its apparent loss.

Perhaps it has to do with the potential for embarrassment, particularly for those who link dignity with bodily control. We are physically exposed to an extent few of us had ever imagined or experienced. Labor in all its intensity moves us to scream and swear and utter things of which we didn't believe ourselves capable. These things happen all the time and shouldn't diminish the dignity of women when they are having a baby. And yet when it comes to maintaining a sense of dignity in birth, the ground upon which childbearing women tread can feel mighty shaky.

Where the ground gets shakiest is in women's assessments of themselves. What we heard time and again from women looking back on birth is that they felt burdened with guilt and shame—with a pervasive sense that they hadn't lived up to an ideal. That by virtue of their birthing mode, choices, or performance, they weren't worthy of others' respect, or of their own. Of her first two births in hospitals, Maisie recollected, "I felt guilty. I didn't want to remember. Just the shame—I don't know," which solidified her resolve to give birth at home. In her first births, as she tells it, she was young and endured disrespectful treatment by hospital staff. Conversely, first-time mom Katha, who gave birth by planned cesarean (her baby had a heart defect that required it), told us that in looking toward her next birth, she felt guilty—like a "wimp"—about her preference to do it the same way again, to have another cesarean—because "the whole goal is to have a natural birth, right?"

So if it seems obvious that respect in birth is important, the women of the Good Birth Project show us that respect is not a simple matter. In this chapter, I cover three ways respect comes up in women's assessments of their births. The first has to do with respect for the event; the second with respect for the childbearing woman and her baby; and the third with how we think about ourselves, and the pervasive problem of shame and guilt.

Respect for Birth

One of the things that makes birth different from other events is that, well, it's *birth*. It's an extraordinary moment in our lives, a turning point. It is respect-worthy, even sacred. Indeed our culture and many others mark pregnancy and birth with what sociologists call *sacralizing* behaviors—ritual practices and beliefs that impart a special status to pregnant women and their experiences of birth. Things that disrupt that status, that understanding of birth as such, can be experienced as traumatic, alienating, disrespectful. Indeed, women tell us that a big part of a good birth is having the people around acknowledge birth's special place in our lives—to pay their respects to birth.

For many women, a good birth means the people in attendance take seriously the notion of birth as major life event. Some compare it to a wedding, highlighting the importance of certain rituals held dear. Wise woman Maisie reflected on what struck her as a failure by her doctor to honor her birth as such with an unceremonious snip of the umbilical cord: "The doctor just cut us apart, like [snaps fingers], 'Oh, oh, did you want to do that? Sorry.' It's almost like saying to a dad, 'Oh, you mean you wanted to walk your daughter down the aisle? Oh, gee, oops.'"

Midwives, for the most part, really get this. Anna, a midwife who works primarily in Latin America attending home births, told us how "honored and privileged" she often feels at "being invited to participate in such a miraculous moment." Plenty of doctors do too, like Colby, who told us how critical she thinks it is to "respect the fact that birth is a very important day in [my patients'] lives and [make] it special for them, and not make it seem like it's just another birth."

For providers, finding ways to make space for meaning is something that often comes with time. Once, in residency, I got bawled out by the attending neonatologist for allowing a father to cut his child's umbilical cord while the neonatology team waited for me to hand them the baby. The neonatologist claimed that the extra ten seconds that meaning-imbued snip took, because it delayed the team's evaluation, had put the baby in harm's way. Of course, it hadn't, but it took a few hundred births for me to know I could push back if ripped at again. There are plenty of us in obstetrics who have found ways to make births celebrated, to help create sacred space within hospital walls and on surgical gurneys, even if doing so is a cultivated skill.

Nevertheless, the dominant cultural narrative is that the place—and even the way—we give birth *does* determine the degree to which it warrants respect. Vaginal births, low-intervention births—these have been hailed as the sorts of births where sanctity is presumed to reside; these are respect-worthy events. With monitors and epidurals, surgeons and scalpels, sanctity will escape us. But as Megan's story suggests, it need not.

Megan, twenty-nine, had her first baby at a community hospital. Like all our first-time moms, we interviewed her before and after birth—and we were fortunate to catch her just days before she delivered. She'd recently gotten the news that her baby was breech and that a cesarean would be the safest route to delivery. She was "extremely disappointed" at first, but by the time we met she said she'd "gotten used to the idea," since scheduling surgery played well with her type-A personality. "I don't consider it ideal," she acknowledged, "but my personality is such that I like knowing when I have to have my laundry done, when the grocery shopping has to be finished. I know exactly what day I'm stopping work." Clearly an optimist, she was looking at a glass half full.

But there was that nagging empty half—that ideal birth had flown the coop. As is the case for many women, with the dissolution of the ideal, Megan's attention shifted. She started thinking about outcome rather than process, and located the good in the reasonable expectation of good health. "It's still going to be a healthy baby, I'm healthy—what more do I want? How picky can I really get?"

What I see in this familiar refrain is the presumption that vaginal birth and meaning are interlaced. When surgery is indicated, something is lost, and the expectation of a birth imbued with meaning is set aside as we refocus on the ultimate reward. "Healthy mom, healthy baby," we tell ourselves; the rest is icing on the cake.

At first glance, this might appear to be a healthy approach, a way to protect ourselves from those dashed hopes and feelings of shame that pervade women's experiences of birth these days. But, I'd counter, that's selling birth short. Birth matters, however we do it. It's the first story in a life, a stage setter, something we will always remember. As sociologist Susan Maushart has put it, birth is a "drama of unprecedented power, not only in the lives of women but in the life of all humanity."

This dampening of expectations, so common among women who hope for a good birth by traditional measures (read: *natural*), is where well-intentioned critiques of hospital birth get us off track. Just because hospital procedures—like the unceremonious snip of an umbilical cord—can feel disrespectful, the sanctity of the event remains. A cesarean is not reason in itself to mourn. As Megan discovered, the orifice through which a baby exits the body doesn't determine whether or not our birth was good, whether or not there is something more to hope for, to expect, than a safe passage to motherhood and the gift of a healthy baby.

Megan's son Liam was born by cesarean as planned on a brisk fall day, just after noon, six and a half pounds, healthy as could be. The birth, Megan told us, was "fantastic . . . an excellent birth experience. It was perfect for us." So good, she told us, she felt lucky to have the option of cesarean for her next child. When we asked her what made it so good, it wasn't just the fact that her sweet boy entered the world, though he was certainly a big part of it. Rather, she found the good in the experience of respect, in the conveyed sense that her birth *did* matter.

> I genuinely felt that they cared about the experience that we had . . . [What made it good] was the respect they had for me and for what I was going through. You talk to someone differently if someone has had, you know, a tonsillectomy versus someone who's just had a baby.

Tricia came to a similar conclusion about what makes for a good birth: having a doctor who was genuinely excited about sharing the moment with her. She'd missed that in her first birth, when her middle-of-the-night labor meant the on-call doctor, her least favorite in the group she'd been seeing, would be summoned out of bed. When Tricia figured out who'd be catching her baby, she thought, "Great, I got the one I didn't want. She's in a bad mood—I'm imposing upon her nighttime rest for her to come deliver my kid."

But Tricia's second birth was a different matter entirely, and it had everything to do with her doctor's recognition of the moment's importance. It wasn't just another procedure, an inconvenience, but a major life event he had the privilege of sharing. Tricia notes:

> There were just little things that happened that made me really appreciate the doctor with this last birth . . . Even in the end he was like, "Now, make sure you get in there and get this

picture—this is the best way to get the picture." He got in the picture and he was taking pictures and was . . . excited to be there for our new baby. He was excited for us and sharing the moment with us, and it wasn't like an imposition for him.

Of course, we can't control how people around us act, and affronts to respect won't be predictably avoidable. But we can do our best to choose providers we think will respect the sanctity of birth, and we can have open conversations about our hopes and expectations, as my patient Suzanne did with me during a clinic visit when she was anticipating her second birth.

I met Suzanne for the first time several years ago toward the end of her pregnancy, on what was a memorably sweltering summer day in North Carolina. Suzanne had by all accounts gracefully managed the third trimester with a toddler in tow, and seemed to be bearing a burden of something other than that thick summer air when I saw her in clinic.

"I need to talk to you about my delivery," she said, flipping pages of a board book for the child who sat on what was left of her lap. "I need you to promise me one thing," she said, with a steely resolve. "Whatever happens, I don't want Dr. Davis anywhere near me. I mean, anywhere."

I was puzzled. I knew from Suzanne's records that her first delivery was absolutely uncomplicated. It began with labor at home, she arrived at the hospital with a nearly dilated cervix, and after two hours of pushing, she delivered a gorgeous, healthy baby boy without a single stitch. She went home the next day. The physician she named, Dr. Davis, was eminently competent, surgically skilled, and at least partially responsible for Suzanne's intact perineum. But then Suzanne told me why she didn't want Dr. Davis in the vicinity. It wasn't about stitches, or brushes with the unthinkable, but it was about an injury of sorts—an injury she was determined to avoid this time around.

Labor had been manageable, Suzanne told me, but by the second hour of pushing, she was losing steam. She'd been up several of the preceding nights with worsening heartburn and a knifelike pain at the center of her pubic bone whenever she turned or had to get out of bed to pee. She was exhausted, and as time crept by, the possibility of cesarean loomed, unmentioned. The nurse, her husband, and the doula cheered her progress, their faces betraying sympathetic pushes of their own with each contraction. It was then that Dr. Davis's words of encouragement—perhaps akin to tough love—struck like daggers: "Come on, Suzanne," she said, "push out this baby, so I can get home in time to read to my kid."

The one thing she had to thank Dr. Davis for, Suzanne told me, was not her unscarred bottom (or her healthy baby, for that matter), but rather that the comment incensed her so completely that she did push her child out, in the midst of what she remembered as a mighty roar. And she never wanted to see Dr. Davis again, especially not in a delivery room.

I tell Suzanne's story not to scare you, but to give a sense of how important these seemingly little things can be—how words can slice through our experiences and memories, especially words that connote some dearth of respect for the monumental event that is, for many of us, birth. I also tell it because I think it is something maternity care providers should hear: Our words matter. We need to be careful about what we say; we need to remember that some of those words will be reified as part of a birth story, a life's beginning, and will shape understandings of whether the experience was good or not. A similar utterance would be unimaginable if the situation were one of dying, rather than birthing. But many of the world's introspective and articulate mothers have linked birth and death, have called them "the same." Understood as such, birth requires not just competence, but respect, reverence.

But how do we secure that? What can we learn from Suzanne? For one, she had an open discussion with me about what she wanted, and I'd encourage those of you who are pregnant to follow her lead looking toward your birth. You can also get a sense of how your doctor or midwife regards birth by talking with them, getting an idea of what they offer and how they approach birth. Do they attend births because obstetrics is "interesting," or because, once they set foot on a labor floor or attended a birth, they were smitten and there was nothing else in medicine they could imagine doing? Look around their clinic space. One of my colleagues from residency—no doubt a birth junkie herself—has a huge bulletin board in her office with snapshots of newborns, quite a few of which are in the arms of the scrub-clad and beaming doctors that caught them. This is a practice full of people who love attending births and relish the opportunity to take part; the bulletin board is evidence of their enthusiasm, of their due regard.

I allow that not everyone wants a doctor or midwife so smitten with birth, and not everyone will get one either. Jess, one of my best—and I'd add most "spiritual"—friends told me that approaching the births of her two children, three things were important: an epidural, a remote (for the TV), and a doctor who'd make sure both were available. But twirling her cappuccino during an afternoon we stole away from our desks—and without a bit of prodding from her birth-junkie girlfriend (me)—she acknowledged the sanctity of birth, how close it is to death. To Jess's thinking, finding that sanctity was a decidedly personal matter; it was up to her, something upon which the arbitrariness that characterizes medical care, even some of midwifery, could not entirely depend.

Indeed, beyond doing our best in our selection of and communication with our providers, even greater certainty can be found in considering the very notion of sacredness and how we might secure it for ourselves. If other people don't acknowledge the sacred in our births, perhaps it is because the sacred in birth is a personal matter—for your birth, *the* sacred is *your* sacred. It is something that can be cultivated and protected, and at its best the sacred will elude the prescriptions upon which the traditional notions of the good in birth have depended.

Nearly seventy-five years ago, sociologist Michel Leiris delivered a now famous lecture titled "The Sacred in Everyday Life." The sacred, he says, can be understood not just in its official or public sense, but as an intensely personal notion that anyone can discover by parsing through the objects and experiences of one's own life—times when we know we are "no longer moving on the level of the ordinary . . . but rather have entered a radically distinct world, as different from the profane world as fire from water." Leiris describes events of his childhood—as mundane as coughing fits of illness, adults speaking in the parlor, watching the jockey at a horse race—which he came to understand as unusual, prestigious, ambiguous, dangerous, breathtaking—and conclusively sacred. In that essay, Leiris takes us through memories and objects that left a resonance of "strong emotion"—things that took his breath away (like racehorses) or struck him as alluringly dangerous (like the coals of a burning hearth fire, which I have observed, firsthand, tug on the impulses in the hearts of little boys) or transformative, as coughing fits that turned the author, imaginative in youth, into "someone of importance—like a tragic hero—surrounded as I was by my parents' worry and loving care."

For many of us, birth is full of objects and moments that have a similarly evocative resonance. As is true of many moms I know, tucked away in my closet is a short stack of the flannel swaddling blankets that pervade hospital nurseries across the United States. I don't use them anymore, but I'd never dispense with them either. When NPR did a story on them, it was hardly surprising (to me) that they received a massive response—more than 2,000 photos of newborns swaddled, often accompanied by intimate, meaning-imbued recollections (not to mention confessions of "smuggling" the blanket home, of holding fast to that sacred linen). One woman interviewed for the story noted that even today the blanket "stirs mixed emotions—overwhelming joy, anxiety, frustration, a sense of incarceration, but mostly . . . the precious bond with a tiny, fragile, lucid human being who became the center of my world." Those blankets—mundane as they are, indiscernible from one another by those of us who use them to wipe off, swaddle the diminutive bodies we help usher in—are imbued with meaning by the mothers who give birth, by the people who become parents, by those for whom the day is perhaps among the sacred in their lives.

No doubt it is helpful to be attuned enough to disruptions (like the one Suzanne endured) in real time, or be accompanied by those who are, and to have the strength, resources, and wherewithal to defend our sacred space. Part of getting to the good in birth is remembering you can say something, and press back if it feels like your sacred is being disrupted. Through birth, women often gain confidence enough to say, "Hey, this is my time, back off, it means something to me." As mother of four Raquel advised, "We feel powerless to be rude to anybody, but I think that women need to feel free to be rude. And not just see it as rudeness, but to say, 'What I need right now is an hour of absolute quiet.'" There are plenty of times in birth when pressing back is not possible, so disruptions won't be entirely avoidable. But to the extent we can speak up, we should.

But what I've also learned is that the sacred will also emerge as time wears on—so it's important to be open to it, to give yourself a chance to sift through your birth (as Leiris did the objects of childhood) and think about what made birth special—to you. My friend Jackie told me after her birth that graham crackers and cranberry juice (which the nurses brought in great supply in the hours and day following the birth) took on a whole new meaning—more like a sacrament than a mere mid-morning snack for toddlers. Midwife Bev told us that for two years after her second birth, when she had trouble sleeping at night, she would "review from the moment I woke up [with contractions] to the moment I had [my daughter]"—a sacred and intensely personal incantation, and one that always restored her sense of calm.

The bottom line is that we can each define our own sacred. When it comes to sacred space, it might be in a home or in a hospital, but sanctity is never out of reach. It's not something that depends on whether a baby is born vaginally or by cesarean, with forceps or a gentle hand. It does, though, require shoring up in the moment of birth, and some attention in the days and months that follow.

Respect for the Childbearing Woman

Many moms also talk about how important it is to be heard, trusted—to be treated as the "experts" when it comes to our bodies or our births. They tell us it's important to surround ourselves with people who will listen, pay attention to what we need and want. No doubt this notion of respect relates back to agency—to being offered choices and being able to decide between them. But respect is also important as an end itself, its implications subtler if no less profound.

Yet in birth this sort of respect can elude us. As implausible as it might seem, as bellies grow and we take up more space, pregnant women all too often become invisible. Not literally, but there's an undeniable pattern of failures to view women as people, of looking past or through us.

My friend Geri, the attorney I introduced in Chapter 1, recalled laboring in an elevator during her second birth as men in suits carried on their conversation about stocks and who was coming to the lunch meeting, as if she weren't there at all, white-knuckling the handrail. Then there is the familiar "public domain of the belly" phenomenon: people reach out and touch our expanding midsections as if they are public property—as if we no longer are their rightful owners, as if we need not be consulted about whether and when the body, our body, is touched, even commented upon. As obstetrician and mother of two Colby put it:

> And they'll talk about you like you're not there. I'd be in the el-evator and people will say, "Oh my God, how many you got in there?" And I'll say, "One." And then they'll turn to each other and say, "Well, she's huge. I can't believe it." And in my head I'm thinking, "You're talking about me like I'm not even here." Or I was getting a pedicure . . . and they proceeded to have a debate on whether or not I should breast-feed. And I'm just like, "Okay, we can talk about the nail color, but not the boobs."

The pattern appears in less public spaces too. For instance, I've noticed that behind closed doors, my colleagues will bat around reasonable options for labor management as if they were their own: "I'd do a cesarean," or "I'd do an amniocentesis," or "I'd do a version," as if the decision to operate, to test, to turn a baby through a woman's abdominal wall was the doctor's alone to make. Of course, these are choices our *patients* face, though their prefer-ences and personhood are pressed away amid our banter, our guidelines, our texts. And as I mentioned in the Introduction, in research and public dis-course, women who are pregnant are all too often treated as "vessels and vec-tors" rather than patients, people in their own right.

Look at me, we want to say, *here I am. I am worthy of your regard. Look.*

I'm not sure why people avert their attention when it comes to pregnancy, to birth. Some might chalk it up to sexism or just gendered ways of attending to women. But more than a few have noticed the same tendency when it comes to dying people, to death. There are certain things that, like the sun, can't be the object of too long, too penetrating a gaze.

It's a point emphasized by many scholars who work on end-of-life issues, who quote La Rochefoucauld's maxim that "death, like the sun, should not be stared at." According to legal scholar Robert A. Burt, we can in fact look at death, but the "prolonged effort will induce a kind of dazzled blindness." I find resonance for this idea with birth, which induces a similar sort of blindness—one in which women and their bodies are erased, respect for their personhood a sudden point of contention.

Kyra, from Chapter 3, was pregnant with her first baby when we initially interviewed her. She had been thinking about birth for years, and now, at thirty-eight, she had a clear idea of what felt right: a birth at home, her favorite place, where she imagined she could feel comfortable and supported. She knew that at home she could spend time in a tub, avoiding medications if possible—a way of life for her and her husband, even out of the context of pregnancy and birth.

Things didn't go quite as planned, though, and on an early August morning after a day of laboring and a cervix that seemed to be stuck at nine centimeters, she agreed at the recommendation of her midwife to be transferred—exhausted, dehydrated—to a hospital. The medevac arrived, and after she walked up her steep driveway, the unexpected happened.

Still laboring hard, Kyra was strapped on her back to a board. Despite the circumstances, Kyra noted that "probably the one unpleasant experience with the whole thing" was her interaction with the paramedic team: "They were questioning me and checking me . . . I told them exactly where I was, and . . . he still pulled my pants down in front of everybody in the ambulance and checked to see if she's crowning."

Kyra knew how dilated she was; she had been stuck at nine centimeters for hours. Her midwife had just confirmed the baby's position moments before. But in failing to engage in either a respectful exchange of words or the simple act of offering to check her with a sheet draped over her knees, the paramedic's behavior was a challenge—in a moment of vulnerability—to Kyra's intellectual and bodily integrity.

For women like Kyra, who elect to deliver babies outside the medical establishment, such exchanges may come up in the process of hospital transfer. Women should plan for them, bracing as if against a wave for interactions with providers who will judge them for their choices—even punish them with unprofessional behavior, like that paramedic did with Kyra. Indeed, none of us are immune to them, wherever we give birth.

This is not to say that this behavior—if deeply unfortunate—is inevitable. Health care providers across the spectrum can and do provide respectful care for women. As our dialogue about birth continues, I think it is unproductive to continue our polarized banter or approach to birth presuming that there are really "two views." Indeed, many of the maternity care providers we interviewed had a more nuanced appreciation of birth, accepted as reasonable the diversity of approaches, the uncertainty that is the endeavor of birth, and the need to respect women in their choices.

I also think it is unproductive to presume, as some birth advocates have suggested, that giving birth in a hospital (whether you choose that setting or are transferred there) will require a fight. As more midwives work in hospital settings and educate medical students, as midwives and doctors partner in developing responsible and patient-centered public policy, as out-of-hospital birth becomes more familiar, I am optimistic about respect, and hopeful that interactions like the one Kyra endured will become more an aberration than ever. And it's an optimism that I think women approaching birth can share.

Indeed, Kyra's story points also to the value of being open to the possibility of respectful care in the context of an evolving birth. Kyra's experience with the paramedic contrasts sharply to her experience in the hospital, where the obstetric team worked with her to facilitate a birth she would still find meaningful and manageable. Again, we see the importance of respect in what Kyra would ultimately make of the birth.

> They really wanted to respect how I wanted to have an unmedicated birth . . . I feel like we conferred with [the nurse] on some level and we decided, "Okay, we'll just try the mini-dose of Pitocin. We don't want to increase it or anything, but let's just . . . see if we can get my uterus to kick in here a little bit more."

Respect can trip up others, even the people we love. Several women in the Good Birth Project recalled going into labor and having their partners question whether their contractions were the "real" thing—some grumbling or turning over in the bed, maybe wishfully thinking that they could clock in a few more hours of sleep before heading off to the hospital. A note to partners: let's just say this doesn't go over well.

Mother of six Jen remembered the "worst thing" about her fifth birth was when her husband didn't believe his (very) experienced wife was in labor.

> The worst thing was that I felt like my husband should call [my midwife]. And he was like, "No, you're not ready." And I was almost in tears. "I am ready. You get her on the phone right now!" I started having contractions and they were pretty regular, but my husband said, "They're really not strong enough and they're kind of irregular. You'll have one at four minutes and then one at six and then not." But I was like, "They are averaging five minutes—you get her on the phone."

It's not just husbands or partners. Mother of four Raquel recalled an experience during her second birth when her epidural wasn't functioning well and she was feeling "everything" on one side. The anesthesiologist had been working on the epidural, trying to tweak it and attributing Raquel's ongoing pain to "some kind of anatomic abnormality." Raquel had been coping, if somewhat miserably, but was assured in the sense that she was being heard and that the persistence of her pain, if "weird," was understood to be real.

But when a new anesthesiologist came on duty, Raquel went from miserable to infuriated when he questioned whether she was "really" in pain.

> Even now I can remember how angry I was at that arrogant fellow who was the anesthesiologist . . . He wouldn't believe me. He kept saying, "I've bloused you [injected medicine into your epidural] as much as I can, and you have a small frame. I just know that it has to be working." And I wanted to rip his head off.

Raquel was still dealing with the same oppressive pain—but this time what she knew (that it hurt!) was questioned, as it didn't seem to "fit" the medical facts.

Even some midwives, steeped in traditions of "trusting women" and "trusting the body," make the mistake. When first-time mom Erica was sure she was laboring—and hard—she told us she too was instructed by her midwife to wait, and found it infuriating. She'd been sent home from the birthing center, and then she called back after several hours.

> I remember [one of the midwives] getting on the phone—
> "Honey, you are not in true labor." I couldn't understand why
> they were telling me this . . . I was so angry that I wouldn't even
> talk to her on the phone. My fiancé had to hold the phone up to
> speakerphone because they wouldn't let me come in until they
> talked to me, and I refused to talk to them because I was in such
> agony and I was so upset. So I just heard that through the speaker-
> phone. "Honey," [laughs] "you need to wait."

I recognize that this all might feel—at first blush anyway—like a hopeless state of affairs. If respect is so important to the good birth, but is essentially out of our hands, what can we do? There is a mountain of lessons for providers here: Be aware of yourself, and what you're scared of. Don't take insecurities out on patients. Don't assume you know what your patient values. Start with congratulations, not apologies. Be compassionate. Be loving. Don't judge. Loved ones too can learn from these stories: your partner or daughter or friend needs you to listen to her, to give her the benefit of the doubt, to support her in what she needs first and foremost. For childbearing women, though, the lessons are less clear-cut, but they exist and they have power.

For one, I think it's helpful to recognize that respect from others *is* out of our hands. We can't orchestrate what other people do or say, which brings us back to that slippery notion of control. Like many of the women of the Good Birth Project, mom of twins Sophie compared her birth and her wedding, both of which she relished, though both had their holes when it came to respect.

> If you are a control freak, I'm sorry. You have to think of it as a
> wedding. You can plan it to the minute, but the day it happens it
> has a life of its own. And it'll just go. You just let it go. Don't get
> mad about it. You know, at my wedding forty people crashed.
> Koreans do that [laughs]. And just go with it. Don't get upset,
> because you have to tell yourself, you've done the best you can.

Second, it's important to understand that other people's reactions to birth and childbearing women are oftentimes a reflection of their own life story more than the one unfolding before them. Birth can bring out the worst and best in people—an anxious paramedic might lash out, compared with the one who is experienced and comfortable, who can refrain from judgment and focus on respectful caring. A nurse might offend in ill-conceived efforts to hide her own insecurities or convey her depth of experience on the labor ward. Doctors, too, bring to birth their own histories, their own births, their own mixture of confidence and fear in the face of birth's uncertainty. As a resident, it took me a long time to feel at ease on Labor and Delivery, to believe that I could walk, not run, that I could and should pause, listen, be open— that the urgency of the event need not diminish my attention to its meaning.

And finally, those disrespectful moments that all too often rivet, if jarring, need not color the whole experience. If every moment of her birth didn't feel respectful, Kyra came to appreciate those that did. Though she didn't have the birth at home she envisioned, she called her birth "a great experience . . . It was great, for how it happened. People were generally . . . respectful and caring. We really accepted that and felt like we would have wanted her at home in the water, into our arms, but the way it happened was fine."

Respect for the Baby

"This is the doctor who helped me have you, honey."

You'd think by now I'd know what to say next when introduced, years after their births, to the children of my patients. It is in fact a thrill to meet them once they are walking and talking and have a sense, however muddled, of their having entered the world through their mother's body.

I'd had the pleasure of attending Millicent's third birth, helping her bring Oliver into the world. His birth reflected his personality—even, steady, lovely, reassuring. But I never understood the depth of Millicent's gratitude until I heard about the births of her other children: Emma, whisked away to the intensive care unit after she came out blue, her umbilical cord wrapped thrice around her neck; and Leo, born pink as could be but with a mass in his abdomen. With Oliver in tow, it was Leo's birth I heard about that morning, when Millicent and I stole a moment to gab among a grocery store's freshly stacked produce.

"I didn't sleep for the first forty-eight hours of his life," recalled Millicent, "because the door kept opening. In would walk another doctor, or resident, or student—wake me up, unwrap my swaddled Leo, and poke and prod his tummy. You couldn't appreciate the mass unless he was crying [making its size and form more obvious], so I started to think they were examining him, hoping he would wake up and cry."

So far, a fairly typical postpartum experience in an academic hospital. Millicent's husband, Doug, had trained in surgery, so they knew pesky residents came with the package.

"Nobody knew what the mass was," she went on. "They were throwing out their best guesses. I remember this one resident, with this filthy white coat, the light brown edges of her sleeves brushing against his face, offering up another possibility for the differential—this tumor, I forget the name, but what I knew from conversations with Doug was that it is devastating, disfiguring, life-ending. And I said, 'I understand that this is very interesting to you, but this is my baby you're talking about.'"

"Did you really say that?" I asked her, thinking she was someone who would.

"No, but that's what I was thinking," she said. "I wish I had."

I have friends in academia who talk about surgery as violence, which always seemed a bit of a stretch to me, attaching more meaning to a necessary abdominal incision than is there, it being part and parcel of an effort to help or cure. But when doctors were sticking needles into my own newborn—and talking about sticking a knife into him on his first day of life, I realized that my friends were onto something.

As I mentioned, William's birth—my fourth cesarean—was respectful in all the ways that I'd hoped for going in. The birth itself was a celebratory event; and as a mother, I felt imbued with due regard. But giving birth to William brought up the importance of respect not just for birth or for the women who do it, but also for the children they bear.

On the second day of William's life, I watched the sun come up and waited for my mother and husband to return and take me back to the space I hated and loved, the intensive care bedside of my newborn. *Hate* is strong word, I know. And there was nothing about my sweet boy to hate. But what I did hate was that he was in that bed, in the unit—far away, poked and prodded by people who I didn't think saw him as the human being he was. People who didn't seem to get the fact that I was a new mother and he was *my baby*.

Initially things were fine, more than fine. The cesarean itself was quite lovely, with none of the drama that characterized his brother's entry into the world, six years earlier. This time I'd handpicked the surgeons, and they did their best work, weaving deftly their twin responsibilities of keeping us safe and making space for the sacred, if surgical, event.

Once William was out and swaddled, the obstetrics team made sure that he and I got our face time before the pediatrics team took him to the intensive care unit for imaging studies—an ultrasound and perhaps an MRI to get a better look at a pesky ellipse in his belly we'd discovered three months prior on a routine sonogram. Those who stayed with me in the operating room kept the sense of occasion alive. I felt like we could have shared champagne.

But then bits started to unravel. I suppose it began just shy of two hours after the last stitch was placed and I was up, with the help of a determined nurse and a large dose of pain medicine, in a wheelchair on my way to the unit to hold my boy.

We were met there with the usual chaos, the hustle and bustle of one of the region's busiest neonatal intensive care units. As we wheeled through, a neonatology fellow I recognized went charging past me: "Where's the kid? Just show me the kid. Get consent for a line. Millie doesn't need to mess with that kid anymore. Get a resident to deal with it." Bruce wasn't exactly known for his restraint, which was perhaps why, according to those who knew him, he felt more comfortable working with humans who couldn't yet talk.

"Geez," I thought. "Must be a busy day here. Good thing the parents didn't hear that." Not for a moment did I think he was talking about my baby. But soon it became abundantly clear he was.

We made our way to William's bedside and found an assembled crowd: surgeons, pediatricians, medical students and residents with clipboards and smartphones in hands—fascinated not by my child's marvelous form but by the mystery of what they couldn't see inside him. I went to get my first real look and there they were, blocking my view and talking about possible diagnoses. My baby, it turns out, was a "great case," a veritable "fascinoma"—a term I'd used myself but now bristled thinking I ever had. The chief surgeon told us that he wanted to order more tests and disclosed that, while they weren't any closer to a diagnosis, Baby Boy Lyerly was on the OR schedule for the end of the day.

I know it can be difficult—especially in moments of vulnerability, when life feels like it is being shaped before your eyes—to know what the right thing to do is, to know whether you should just give in to the experts or listen to your intuitions. I struggled with it, frantically and silently, on William's first day, and Kim and I are both doctors, admittedly with more knowledge and authority than most others who will face similar situations in birth. But I will say that what moved me eventually to act on my intuitions and raise objections to what the medical team proposed to do stemmed in large part from my sense that we were not being given due regard, that we were not seen as mother and child, that William was not being adequately respected. Without such, it was unimaginable to me that anyone could know what was best for us. I eventually took it to be the silver lining of disrespect: it provided me with a steely resolve to question the team's reasoning and pursue other options—a wait-and-see approach instead of surgery, which gave us just the reprieve and information we needed (more on this later). It is not just that disrespect feels bad; it is a clue that you should raise questions, press back, or get someone by your side who will.

Fortunately, there is not always a serious medical decision under consideration (no doubt I'd trade my silver lining any day), and lack of due regard is not always a sign that medical decision-making is askew. Sometimes the offense is all there is. Indeed, none of us likes to feel like a medical object, whatever the situation. Familiar to many are accounts of how being reduced to "a case" or—even worse—a body part by medical staff can be experienced as an offense at best, an offense whose poignancy is redoubled in the setting of birth. But if many of us arrive at birth with thick enough skin to deflect impersonal treatment of ourselves, treatment of our new children as objects feels nearly unforgivable. Our babies have just found their way into existence and intimations that they are less than fully people strike us as unfathomable, as threatening as the specter of death itself. I will say that I identified so intensely with my children that I found it hard, at times, to distinguish their pain—their very existence—from my own, especially when they felt freshly pulled over life's edge.

The wrong words can stick—for years. Karla, a grand multipara (indeed, a mother of seven), recalled a comment by a nurse during her sixth birth—a first girl after five boys.

> I never will forget this. It was kind of derogatory. She said, "How do you think you can get this split-tail out?" And I remember not knowing what a split-tail was and I said to my husband, "What is a split-tail? Why do they keep saying that?" You know, there was a nurse saying that, just an old Southern saying I guess that meant a female child. I'm like, "Why is she calling my female child a derogatory name that's in my uterus?" [laughs] You know, give me a break. So that stuck out for me.

Karla had been through birth seven times when she told us this story—if anyone had a chance to develop thick skin, she did. But with layers of experience, what crystallized for Karla was that respect and words matter. They mark a birth, and a life. They can disrupt sacred space. They endure. "People depend on your humanism," she offered as advice to those of us who attend birth. "If you are not willing to be humanistic, perhaps you need to do something else." I couldn't agree more.

Of course, we can't control what other people do and say about the baby, and that's one of the difficult things about respect. Usually it is something bestowed by others. And not everyone will know how to show it, or be moved to do so, and it is certainly something those of us who care for women in birth need to get better at. It should be lesson one, day one of training, in my view. But I think it is important to consider the lessons women tell us they've learned from their experiences.

For one, providers won't always know when they've crossed a line; as we've seen, in birth what is sacred can be an entirely personal matter. When my friend Jackie's obstetrician came to check on her after her second cesarean, she oohed and aahed, then used the baby's name, to Jackie's immediate dismay. Her parents were in the room, and she had not yet announced outside the operating room the name she had chosen. "My doctor was mortified," she recounted, "when she realized her transgression." Ack, I thought, wondering (as I tend to) how many times I must have crossed a similar line, created a similar wrinkle in an unfolding birth story.

"But you know, Annie," Jackie said, perhaps sensing my worry, "I love my doctor, so it didn't matter to me in the end, really. I knew by then that I had no control of stuff like that. But I trusted her intentions, so it was okay."

And I know I have been given a pass or two myself. Gabe, a research colleague of mine, has reminded me (and a good many of our mutual acquaintances) of one of my classic missteps, taken while caring for his wife and newborn several years back. In advance of circumcising their new baby, I was explaining the procedure, describing for Gabe and his wife, Jody, that I'd inject a bit of anesthesia before beginning—assuring them (to their initial confusion and enduring amusement) that "It's just a little prick"—referring to the injection of numbing medicine.

"Indeed it is," Gabe replied with a chuckle—the allusion to a different sort of prick, lost on no one but their earnest and perhaps sleep-deprived doctor.

Of course, all transgressions are not so forgivable, but are worth considering in context: they most often stumble across the lips of someone who wants what you do in birth—an event that is satisfactory in both process and end.

Ultimately, we can't orchestrate respect from others—and especially not in birth. What we can do is attend to the value of respect when it's conveyed and what it tells us about the nature of care we are receiving, and not take it personally when respect is absent. I think about its occasional absence as an off-color string (even a snag) in the tapestry that makes up a birth story that, as a whole, over time, we can come to embrace. While we might not have the power to change how things are happening in the moment, we can control how we think about them afterward. But perhaps the most important caveat remains: we can sometimes be our own harshest critics.

Taking the Reins: Self-Respect

I had this complete acceptance for how things happened outwardly, but it wasn't there for my own performance. I felt like . . . I just let myself get in the way.

—KYRA

I don't know what it is about the grocery store—it seems to be a place where people feel free to talk about all manner of experiences pertaining to birth. It is where Millicent unloaded about Oliver (and I, to her, about Will). I can't begin to count the number of conversations I've had amid pyramids of oranges and rows of cereal boxes. But these are the spaces where conversations, for better or for worse, seem to erupt.

Some, inevitably, are for worse. When we women talk about birth, public spaces become forums not just for helpful mirroring, but for judgment, fertile ground for cultivating guilt and shame. At a postpartum visit, a patient of mine described an incident at a local organic grocery store. With newborn strapped to her chest, she was sorting through the best produce North Carolina had to offer. A stranger approached her and asked—perhaps innocently—about her recent birth and whether she had used the local freestanding birth center.

When the woman learned my patient had given birth at the hospital, with an epidural, she took a step back and said, "Oh, I'm sorry, that must have been awful." It wasn't, she insisted, recounting the incident to me, but she hadn't been able to shake the sense that there was something she missed out on, something for which she could be pitied, of which she should be ashamed, by virtue of the choices she'd made about delivering her son.

All too often, birth becomes a source of judgment and shame. What I was dismayed to find in talking to women of the Good Birth Project was that the most important arbiter of respect—oneself—ends up doubting most whether it is deserved.

For one thing, birth for many women involves unprecedented "public" exposure. As Karla put it, "Women do feel vulnerable, taking off your clothes in an office or hospital, and spreading your legs and you're having a baby." Given what birth requires, women can feel ashamed of their bodies, even when those bodies are doing extraordinary things.

But bodies aren't the only thing that birth exposes. In birth we are often pushed to our limits, and so we can feel exposed in other ways. Our mettle, the extent of our patience, our tolerance for pain and uncertainty are all tested. If our bodies are exposed to varying degrees, so is our character, so are our souls. As such, birth can make women feel ashamed of themselves—for how they acted, what they were able to accomplish, what giving birth seemed to reveal about who they are and of what they are made.

Exposure may be a given, but shame is not.

Take the question of nakedness. Stephanie described herself as a "modest" person ("I don't even wear bikinis"). But when she got pregnant with triplets, her doctors recommended cerclage, a stitch placed around the cervix to help keep the babies inside. The procedure is done in the operating room under regional anesthesia, meaning the patient is awake but numb. It is high-stakes, delicate, and it requires lots of eyes and helping hands holding retractors and passing instruments. For Stephanie, it would mean stirrups and waist-down exposure for considerably longer than the usual—unnerving if tolerable—pelvic exam. But getting a cerclage, although a harrowing prospect to modest Stephanie, turned out to be remarkably unproblematic, her dignity unshaken.

Part of it, she said, had to do with how people in the operating room treated her. Nobody else was fazed; they acted like it was just "ordinary that they see women in these positions all the time." The staff was respectful but also "oblivious in some sense that [nakedness] was even an issue. And that it was fine. I think that probably made me feel less self-conscious that they were like 'This is no big deal.'"

But part of the reason Stephanie left the cerclage with her dignity intact had to do with how she saw herself. As uncomfortable as it was to be splayed and gazed at for the better part of an hour, she felt she was exposed for a reason—a good reason in her book. And with that she pressed any indignity of exposure firmly to the side.

At some point you just feel like this is what you have to do for your kids. Like this is what being a mom is all about. You are going to do things that make you very, very uncomfortable and that you never, ever do. It's just one of those sacrifices.

Whether or not you think sacrifice is part and parcel of virtuous mother-hood, what Stephanie's experience shows is that how we feel about ourselves and how we feel about our births are not totally out of our hands. Rather, it's a complicated mixture of how others see us and how we see ourselves; whether we are living up to other people's standards and whether we are liv-ing up to our own. Stephanie found dignity not just through the respectful comportment of strangers working between her legs, but also from an evolv-ing sense of what that experience meant to her.

For some women, pregnancy can be refreshingly liberating to the extent that it allows them to dispense with some particularly shame-engendering cultural ideals. The pressure to be model-thin, for instance, gets put aside, and many pregnant women are happy to embrace the idea that curves, even fat, are evidence of responsible, empowered, respect-worthy living. Though as sales of the iconic *What to Expect* indicate, the tug of shame during preg-nancy is plenty forceful. "Before you close your mouth on a forkful of food," author Murkoff advises, "consider 'Is this the best forkful of food I can give my baby?'" and women are left to mull, regret, and try to justify that mouth-ful of carrot cake that simply gave them pleasure the evening before.

If the "musts and mustn'ts" of pregnancy are guilt-inducing, birth itself can bring even more oppressive mantras. For instance, there is a broad sense that a good birth is one in which women are in control of *themselves*—with the right breathing techniques, the perfect birth ball and attendant, or a well-placed epi-dural, they can give birth with self-possession and calmness, they can maintain their composure, they can preside over their births with a certain gravitas.

For some women, dignity really does have to do with composure, and plenty of women talked about wanting to be calm—to refrain from screaming or swearing, from hurling angry words at the people in attendance. It's a reason some women give for getting an epidural, and it's a source of pride for women who maintain an appearance of calm without one. For example, Wren told us:

> I didn't want to scream, I didn't want to yell. I wanted to be very
> ladylike about the whole birthing process . . . I didn't want to

blame my husband—you know it takes two. I remember I did say "shit" once, but that was it. I maintained my dignity and I just grunted like I had to get it out, but that was it. I was proud of myself for that too.

But like many women, Maisie found she couldn't find that calmness—during her first birth, she screamed and swore and did what "felt good at the time." But it didn't feel good the next day, and led her to compare the experience to a drunken night on the town.

You wake up the next morning and go, "Oh my God, what did I do?" To look back on your birth experience and to suddenly feel ashamed and embarrassed—every time you look back, it's not with joy, you don't want to relive it . . . You're around people you don't know and sometimes you even catch them looking at you a certain way, and you're wondering why. Just like, they made me feel so ashamed for screaming.

For her second birth, Maisie tried keeping quiet. "I didn't make a sound," she noted. But she felt judged for other things, like her decision to eschew an epidural in a hospital where epidurals were routine. So for her third birth, she decided to stay home. There, she told us, she could finally be "herself"—shielded from the imposing gaze of strangers.

What Maisie discovered over the course of her births was that there isn't a universal formula to maintaining dignity in birth—that image of the quiet and restrained woman didn't align with her needs, didn't align with *her*. It was other people who felt unnerved, uncomfortable with screaming, nakedness, full-bore Maisie. Ultimately, where she found dignity was in the privacy of her home, where she could be true to herself in birth.

Other mantras can be equally guilt-inducing—like those that link the "good" with the degree to which a birth is "natural"—or not. If Maisie felt judged for eschewing the epidural, countless others feel judged—and judge themselves—for using one. Bev, a midwife, had tremendous guilt about her first birth, though she and her baby were physically unscathed. She did nothing to be ashamed of, but labor with heart and soul. Yet, exhausted after nearly a day of hard contractions, she got an epidural and delivered vaginally with forceps: "As a midwife, unmedicalized birth was the norm—you know I felt like such a failure."

Perhaps it is no wonder. If epidurals are at the ready inside most hospitals, many women face considerable pressure outside their walls to give birth without the help of that inimitable catheter. The very notion of "natural" and its positive valence is wrapped up with rejection of pain medicine—as if delivering a baby vaginally with analgesia is somehow "artificial" and thus less respect-worthy. Natalie, introduced in Chapter 2, worried while pregnant that getting an epidural would make her feel like she "had a baby but didn't really have a baby." She assured us it didn't when she was actually giving birth, but that assurance comes up against a broad notion that getting an epidural is somehow a cop-out, or a complication. Indeed, countless publications group epidural and analgesia use along with maternal and neonatal morbidity as "adverse" outcomes. The message to mothers? Good ones endure the pain.

It is no wonder that self-respect is under fire in birth. It was hard to miss, over the course of the Good Birth Project, a sort of awe reserved for women who manage to deliver without an epidural or other analgesia. I myself had a considerable amount of awe for Kyra, who—by her own volition—endured an extensive vaginal repair (by an OB she described as "not that gentle"), aided only by a towel between her teeth and the reassuring words of her husband. In fact, that awe was the reason my research team and I decided to jettison our original plan to interview some women for the Good Birth Project in groups—when one, but not all of the interviewees delivered without analgesia, there was an unproductive deference among the others.

It's not just about being a good mother, though. What came through in several interviews was that eschewing an epidural has something to do with being hard-core and tough, capable, a good woman. Time and again, women who gave birth without an epidural talked about how empowering it was, how "impressed with themselves" they are, how the experience made them feel like they could do "anything." Mother of two Martha, who labored so quickly in her second birth that she ended up delivering on her kitchen floor, reflected:

> Everywhere I go, people know me as the woman who had the
> child on the kitchen floor . . . It made me feel like a strong per-
> son, to think, "If I could endure that, I can endure anything . . .
> If I could give birth without drugs and feel that pain, I can do
> this, or I can do that." So I guess it gave me more confidence.

I have no doubt that unanesthetized labor can empower. It's certainly
something to embrace, to make space for, to ensure is an option for those
who desire it (more on this in Chapter 7).

But here is the rub: there is a difference between clearing space for choice
and advocating a single option as superior. All too often, the mantra of empowerment slips and becomes a vehicle for judgment. "I always hear people
that had epidurals feeling like they really missed out," reflected Amanda, a
first-time mom who had the birth she hoped for in a birth center. "I never felt
at any point in time in the labor that I wanted something to ease the pain. I
kind of experienced it all, and I kind of earned him, if that makes sense."
Where, one wonders, does that leave everyone else?

All too often, it leaves them pressing guilt aside—some more success-
fully than others. Take first-time mom Katha, for example, introduced in
Chapter 4. If anyone understands pain with purpose, it is she—just five years
before she gave birth to Nate by cesarean, she was a world-class swimmer at
the top of her game. But birth didn't seem to her to be a place where she
wanted or needed to test her body or mettle. It was about getting her baby
out safely, swiftly, and perhaps most to the point, comfortably. But inevitably
she wavered in her certainty:

> From what I experienced and the whole moment that was so
> easy, really, I feel like, why would I want to go through that la-
> bor pain if I didn't have to? But at the same time, it's still really
> hard on my body and I have a giant scar and things like that.
> Still, I feel like a little bit of a wimp with the fact that I say I'd do
> [a cesarean] again.

Yet in the end, Katha found respect in the extraordinariness of having
gestated a child, rather than her ability to grind through the pain of birth.

I think I feel still pretty amazing—it's pretty amazing that there's a baby that can come out of there. That was in my stomach and that grew, and it sort of makes you realize how amazing the female body is.

Katha's thoughtful reflection brings up another notion—well intentioned, but I think at the heart of the shame that has plagued women time and again. It is the idea, advanced powerfully by midwife Ina May Gaskin, that the female body is "designed" to give birth. "Your body is not a lemon!" she writes reassuringly at the end of her book, *Ina May's Guide to Childbirth*, in which she explains how she has achieved remarkably low rates of cesarean and instrumental delivery. Gaskin's work is a source of guidance for maternity care providers and a source of inspiration for a huge number of women approaching birth. But it is also at the heart of shame that rattles so many women whose births don't go as planned.

Such was the case for Kyra, who hoped to give birth at home but ended up with a vaginal birth in a hospital setting. By all accounts, the birth was magnificent—she was magnificent. Nevertheless, the insistence of the midwifery community on the functionality of the female body and the promise of ecstasy in birth weighed on Kyra. She found it hard to shake an emerging sense of shame and concluded that she had only herself to blame for not having the birth she'd hoped for or envisioned—that birth at home, overlooking the Pacific. "I would never say it wasn't a good birth . . . If there was any part of it that wasn't . . . good, it was that part that had to do with myself." She went on to reflect:

In the days and weeks after, what I felt like was that I didn't do a good job. That was what kept coming up—"I didn't labor well with her," and I felt like . . . I let myself get in the way. And everybody was just, "You did great. You did great." But I never felt like I did great. I really felt like I struggled and that it wasn't graceful. The inner critic was just raging [laughs], as far as how I did.

I really had to process that side of the birth and how I perceived myself in it, and if I thought that there was any part of it

that wasn't . . . good, it was that part that had to do with myself.
And how I perceived myself dealing with it.

Mother of two Molly had the same feelings of disappointment and was
equally critical of herself. After a long labor at the birth center, she was transferred to the hospital in hopes that an epidural and a bit of Pitocin could move
her labor along, but she never dilated past seven centimeters. Ultimately, she
underwent cesarean and delivered a healthy baby boy, but nevertheless felt as
if she "failed."

> I felt like a failure. Maybe my expectations were just too high? I
> don't know . . . But yeah, I was like the biggest advocate for nat-
> ural birth, and I was the only one in our Bradley class that ended
> up with a C-section. It was depressing. The whole time you have
> all these doubts—"Well, what did I do wrong, or what could we
> have done differently?"

"You did nothing wrong," I'd tell her. But guilt from a cesarean can be
hard to avoid, especially with the drumbeat of caution, concern, and judgment that surrounds it. A few years back, highly publicized reports of women
choosing cesarean for their first birth—reasonably, on many fronts—met
with accusations that such women were "too posh to push."

Women like Molly also have to contend with reports linking cesarean
birth with health problems in children, such as the recent one questionably
positing a correlation between cesarean birth and childhood obesity. "If I'd
only been tougher, or more relaxed or thinner," too many women think, "my
child would have been better off."

This is, of course, the wrong conclusion. It's not just that most of these
studies have flaws, but the efforts to reduce cesarean are in large part public
health efforts—blunt instruments to shift behavior across populations. And
it's important to understand that there are many reasons for such efforts, not
all of which are relevant to individual women. For some concerned policy
makers, the driver is economics; for others the worry is that high cesarean
rates will further reduce access to low-intervention birth—if reasonable
concerns, neither has a place in women's assessment of themselves. Perhaps

the most powerful driver is the presumption that there is a "right" or "ideal" way to give birth. But what we know from the women of the Good Birth Project is that this is far from the case.

Few dispute that there are too many cesareans—some are done for the wrong reasons, like fear of liability, or just plain fear, and those are the ones we should avoid. But cesareans can be lifesaving; a world without access to them would be a scary place to give birth. Indeed, I am grateful that, if push comes to shove, I can get a stuck baby out of a woman's body quickly and safely—that in the hospital I have what it takes to save a life, or two.

This invoking of blame is, to be sure, a potential danger of any shared notion of what is desirable in birth. One might worry that it is a potential danger of the Good Birth Project itself, as it proposes a new conception— women-centered though it is—of what makes for a good birth. If we can't live up to it, the worry goes, it too might propagate the very guilt and shame that it aims to eliminate.

But listening to women makes me worry less about that. Not all the women we interviewed fell prey to the blame game, and their stories are a source of wisdom for those of us who have had a harder time shaking it off. All of them, it turns out, ended up embracing deeper notions of the "good" that emerge time and again, whatever the birth mode or its distance from what they had imagined, before birth, as ideal.

Natalie, who gave birth first without an epidural, then with one, said she felt "smarter" the second time around, and talked about meaning she found in birth because of (not in spite of!) an epidural. And Raquel told us, "I really feel like my cesarean was every bit as positive as any of my other [vaginal] deliveries, if not my best delivery." Giving birth more than once, more than one way, helped Natalie, Raquel, and many others figure out what mattered most to them, and they emerged unapologetic for their choices and experiences.

First-time mom Carol also held guilt at bay with certainty that is inspiring. Recall she'd set her heart on an out-of-hospital birth. But after laboring all night at home, her midwife realized that the baby was breech (bottom down) and beyond what she felt safe managing outside the hospital. Like Kyra, Carol had a bad interaction with a judging health care provider but pressed back with ferocity.

There was this nasty nurse, the first person I interacted with, who started to tell me, "Well, this is why you should have gotten a sonogram right before you went into labor, and you shouldn't try to do this at home." And I just railed at her. I said, "I do not need a lecture from you on this right now." I was mean—I was really annoyed at her. And I told her how I felt.

What was most notable to me, though, was the way that she pressed any *self-blame* aside. She felt good about her birth because she felt good about *herself.* When we asked her how she felt about having a cesarean—about not getting the sort of birth she'd been sure was hers to have, there wasn't a whiff of guilt.

I feel good. Yeah. I feel good about it. I feel like I did everything I could to have . . . a birth that wasn't taken away from me by everybody else. I felt like it was still my experience, my family's experience.

Carol could look back on her birth with the sense that medical intervention was necessary for a safe passage. Her birth wasn't ruined because it wasn't what she envisioned. Rather, it was good because it was her very own—nobody "took it away" from her.

Megan, too, who delivered Liam by cesarean, felt great about her birth—not just because it went smoothly or because of the respect she got from others, but because she realized just how much she had done to make it happen.

I'm pretty proud of myself! It's amazing what I can do! You feel guilty about everything as a mom. Like, "Did I do that right?" But I think I'm a more confident person now than I've ever been. I'm pretty proud of myself and, you know, I've got this really healthy, happy baby. Everything he's needed in life he's gotten from me— love and care and food. So I'm pretty proud of myself.

Even Liz, whose second birth didn't go smoothly at all, found self-respect in the tenacity required to endure that birth's disappointments. If her first

birth—a good one, by her account—was satisfying, her second, "very negative" birth made her feel stronger and boosted her confidence.

> You feel like, if you can do that, you can do basically anything. I
> think it makes you feel more powerful, more self-assured . . .
> When you're done with it, you look back and you're just like,
> "Wow, I did that?" That's pretty amazing, that you can create
> life.

Not everyone will make peace with their births so readily, but the process may be its own reward. For Kyra, the good in birth was ultimately not in
the timing or place, and not just in the safe passage, but also in the wisdom
that ensued.

> Now I feel a lot kinder towards myself. It's kind of a life lesson
> for me, being able to accept what goes on with myself as much as
> I accept what goes on outside of myself.

A wise woman, indeed. It is a lesson that will no doubt serve during the
challenges of motherhood. As my mom has reflected and reassured me countless times in the past decade, "We do the best we can do, Annie. And angels
can do no more."

six

Knowledge

The majority of women, literate or illiterate, come to childbirth as a charged, discrete happening: mysterious, sometimes polluted, often magical, as torture rack or "peak experience." Rarely has it been viewed as one way of knowing and coming to terms with our bodies, of discovering our physical and psychic resources.

—ADRIENNE RICH

I have always been extremely fond of the definition of Death which says it is: Inaccessibility of Experience, a Jamesian view, but so good. And for a woman to be deprived of the Great Experience her body is formed to partake of, to nourish, is a great and wasting Death.

—SYLVIA PLATH

I have mentioned a time or two over the course of this book a "mysterious ellipse"—a dark shadow detected in William's belly before he was born. Funny thing, after all the head scratching (and perinatal tussling), the ellipse turned out to be a "lympho-vascular malformation." Sounds bad, I know. But as Kim has been quick to point out ever since we zeroed in on the diagnosis, it is actually a birthmark of sorts, in the family of port wine stains that get children asking questions of each other in swimming pools, that we forget to notice once we know the person whose body they grace. And if it had shown up on the outside of William's body on the day of his birth, rather than on the inside via an ultrasound screen weeks before, the hand-wringing it inspired would have been of an entirely different sort. No doubt our glimpsing it in utero shaped Will's birth in many ways, and threatened to disrupt my grasp on things about birth I had come to recognize as good.

What I haven't mentioned is that our seeing the ellipse in the first place was a well-intentioned mistake, the result of looking when nothing pressed us to, save ready access to fancy machines and a sense of caution given my age and reproductive history. I'd had all the recommended scans. This one was extra, just in case, and that was fine with me, at the time. I had chosen a cautious obstetrician on purpose. I wanted her to be careful, obsessive, and she took the lead. "Let's just look, Annie," I remember her saying, "to make sure he's growing"—despite my new stretch marks that indicated, no doubt, that he was.

My doctor didn't have to twist my arm. Far from it. I've always loved ultrasounds, the chance to glimpse inside, have my breath stolen. Some feminist theorists say ultrasounds alienate women from their own ways of knowing, from "embodied knowledge," but I have always regarded those black-and-white images as an enhancement to knowledge, unarguably moving and reassuring too.

Yet William's mid-trimester scan proved to be something else entirely. It worried us all. It led to more tests, the heavy hand of a pediatric surgeon in the course of our postpartum hospital stay, concern as well as delight marking his brothers' first meeting with him, an IV catheter in his brand-new arm, the strain on connectedness I mentioned in Chapter 4, and continued conversations and worries to press away during his first year of life.

The women of the Good Birth Project tell us that information is important to a good birth. When I asked midwife Kitty Ernst what she thought made for a good birth, "information" was the first thing she offered—perhaps thinking back to the days when it was a rare commodity, when women approached birth knowing very little about their gestating bodies or the process of birth ahead.

But as my recent experience with Will attests, information has a *valence*. Sometimes it is immensely valuable. Other times, it can mislead, can get us off track, can harm us even when it comes in the form of a welcome test or conversation. To boot, there is no way to know everything. I've continued to learn through the course of my life, through my experiences as a student, a resident, an attending doctor, a researcher, a friend, a mother and daughter.

There is so much information these days—and of variable quality—it can be hard to know where to start and whom to believe.

If this seems like a hopeless or overwhelming state of affairs, it's not. Again, women's voices help clear the way and illuminate the ways in which knowledge is important.

In this chapter, I'll talk about the three ways women say knowledge can be in service of the good birth. First is preparation: knowing enough about birth going into it that it's not scary, that there is a familiarity about what is happening to your body, that you've done some informed deliberating about things that might matter to you. But the sort of preparation that makes a difference is not (as midwives and doctors who have given birth can attest) about having a command of the obstetrics or midwifery literature; nor is it about being certain of what you want. That sort of knowledge will take us only so far, and it's important to be careful not to put too much stock in one view, one approach, one particular idea about how birth is or should be. In thinking about planning for birth, and the ever-fraught concept of the "birth plan," wise women tell us that flexibility is key. And certainly part of getting a grasp of things on the front end—of reading up, whatever your source—is the humility that often accompanies the accumulation of knowledge.

Second, the knowledge that women value also relates to communication, especially during birth. They speak of the importance of understanding in real time what is happening and why. Birth feels different from how most of us imagine it, and oftentimes our need to know things exceeds our ability to do so. A drama is unfolding and we are on the stage, perspective is lost, and we hunger for a view from the orchestra—or a well-regarded critic's discerning narrative.

And third, there is the knowledge of experience. Indeed, what was true for many of our wise women was that their births got better and better over time. It wasn't that they had more time to scour the literature on birth. Instead the demands of motherhood meant that they had much less time—no more sitting on the couch with a stack of pregnancy how-to books or poring over the mommy blogs. Having a baby, going through birth, pulled them away from the usual conceptions of what makes birth good, and they had a chance to craft—and then pursue—a notion of the good that was their very own.

Knowledge and Birth

It might be said again that it's obvious—that of course knowledge is important to a good birth—it's important in all manner of situations: when you are buying a house, deciding whom to marry, and, of course, when you are making decisions that bear in some way on your health or the health of your child.

But as psychologists, economists, and others point out, more information is not always better. Too many choices can paralyze us. The way options are presented can have an impact on what we decide to do, sometimes driving us away from what we really want or what is most beneficial to us; and certain information can be irreparably unnerving. However, the right information, from sources ranging from textbooks to experienced moms, can reduce anxiety and clear the path to the good. The trick is figuring out what information that is. It's challenging, to say the least.

For one, women often approach information about birth in the context of the birth wars—heated debates among professionals and advocates about the contours of U.S. maternity care. In this setting, it can be difficult to know whom to trust and what to take from the research that's out there. I've already spilled plenty of ink, for instance, on the debate about the safety of out-of-hospital birth, and it is just one of many contested areas. Indeed, approaches to maternity care are vigorously disputed. The American College of Obstetricians and Gynecologists (ACOG) publishes well-referenced and carefully crafted guidelines and recommendations for practice, at which advocates of midwifery take aim, claiming lack of analytic scope or rigor or, even more commonly, conflict of interest. For instance, a newsletter posted on the website of Citizens for Midwifery, a consumer-based organization that promotes midwifery care, notes, "We've learned to mistrust ACOG largely because our experience has shown that some of their information is inaccurate or self-serving." No doubt there is and will likely continue to be some degree of tension between obstetrics and midwifery, but when guidelines and recommendations are the subject of debate, childbearing women can feel unsure about where the truth lies.

Complicating matters, whatever the alliance, is that the evidence upon which maternity care is based has historically lacked rigor. This is the second reason knowledge is so hard to get a handle on when it comes to birth, and is worth going into in some detail. There are some persistent and gaping holes in our knowledge about pregnancy and birth. Many are due to reluctance to enroll pregnant women in research studies, or the impracticability (and improbability) of signing up women in randomized studies of two very different birth options (like birth inside and outside the hospital). And much of the time in obstetrics, research happens retroactively—*after* an intervention has already made its way into general practice.

Consider medication use. Anyone who provides maternity care will tell you that pregnant women and their spouses and loved ones (as well as doctors in other specialties) continuously press the question of whether certain medications are safe in pregnancy. The honest answer is almost always "Probably, but we don't know." Most medications used during pregnancy have not been tested (and are not approved for use) in pregnant women.

One response is to just presume medications are risky and avoid them all—what I call the "Don't take it, don't use it, don't do it" mentality that pervades thinking about pregnancy. But the truth is that it's dangerous to just go off all medication during pregnancy. Plenty of studies show that failing to treat medical illness during pregnancy can have serious and immediate consequences for pregnant women and their babies. What this means is that the optimal course of action—the right medication, the right dose, the right timing—is in the best circumstances uncertain, and all too often anyone's guess.

So responsible doctors and midwives will do their best to *assure*, but they can't *insure*. When I offer or recommend a treatment to a patient, I believe in my heart of hearts it's safe or, all things considered, beneficial and am more than willing to review what is known about it and how I came to the conclusion I did. But I've found that the fact that I've taken something myself (like a reflux medication) during one or more of my pregnancies is often more assuring to women than the stack of papers I can pull for them.

In some areas of medicine, evidence has improved over the years. In 1979, Archie Cochrane, a famous British epidemiologist, gave obstetrics the "wooden spoon award" as the least scientific specialty in medicine. Since then, research has surged and many obstetric interventions previously assumed to be valuable have emerged as useless or harmful. The best of evidence is now catalogued in the massive Cochrane Database, which systematically collects and parses research on a breadth of topics in medicine, distilling it for doctors and patients alike.

But ready access to this database (or any other) will take you just so far. For one, it's massive. There are more than 700 reviews pertaining to pregnancy alone, each of which represents a distillation of the best research on a fairly narrow issue. And despite the volume, your question might not be captured in the research that's been considered feasible or rigorous enough to be included. Finally, even when research is done well, we all need help getting a sense of how it relates to *us*, even when we completely comprehend the data.

Many years ago, I realized how true this was. Pregnant with Charlie, I watched in horror as my second son, Paul (then not quite two years old), did a face-plant on our kitchen floor, knocking his front tooth nearly out. He eventually developed an infection in the root of the tooth, and his dentist offered us two options: pull the tooth or do a root canal. He reviewed in great detail the options and the studies that supported both as reasonable and safe. But I had no idea what to do until I got a second opinion. In addition to describing the very same facts, that second dentist offered context: "We can do the root canal—it can be fairly involved—or we can pull the tooth. It takes a few minutes, and boys are often pleased with their new 'whistle hole.'" Let's just say Paul's toothless smile was a trademark of Lyerly photos until his adult tooth grew in, five years later. As I said, numbers can take you just so far; then you need someone to help you figure out what they mean, *to you*.

What this means is that you need someone to help give context to numbers, to give you a sense of how to understand them in relation to your body, your pregnancy, what you value, your hopes about or reflections on your experience of childbirth. There is a lot of information at our fingertips, but finding someone—usually a midwife or doctor—who can distill it, provide a frame and a bit of wisdom, is where empowerment through information resides. And when you find someone, you still have to listen to them with the caveat that they may be entrenched in the birth wars, and that their view of the good birth will not always coincide with your own. But without someone to provide some context, it's easy to feel overwhelmed by information overload.

The third and final reason that sifting through information is so difficult is that, even outside the context of the birth wars, different people have different ideas about what counts as valuable or empowering information. Indeed, whatever its health implications, technology is seen by some people as a threat to knowledge itself. Technology's critics argue that it usurps women's authority, undermines us as the experts: We used to "know" when our babies moved, and now we rely on an ultrasound to tell us that information. We used to "know" when we were in labor, but now a monitor strapped to our belly tells us when we are contracting and when we aren't.

But oftentimes women don't see things this way. If technology is sometimes a threat, more often it really is a source of knowledge—it tells us things we want to know. When my friend Chloe faced the threat of preterm labor, she found great solace in a medical test that told her that her contractions were of the Braxton-Hicks variety—that they did not in fact signal early labor. The few patients I've cared for who have suffered a stillbirth in a prior pregnancy often value, and highly, what an external monitor or ultrasound will tell them when they are pregnant again—that their baby is alive and vigorous. These instruments give them a reprieve—however brief—from the embodied vigilance that otherwise characterizes their final weeks of pregnancy, the vigilance some feel they somehow failed at in a prior pregnancy, when a baby died inside them.

Tonya talked about the value of technology when she reflected on her first birth, which was complicated by hemorrhage early in the third trimester.

> I felt like [technology] was very useful during my pregnancies. I can't imagine going to the emergency room and there being no ultrasound machine, and going through what I went through with [my daughter] and not knowing why I am bleeding like this— without the use of the ultrasound they would not have been able to see that it was my placenta that was low-lying . . . [With] the advancements in technology and medicine, they were able to immediately give blood to me and have me transfused . . . I can't do anything but say that [technology has] been wonderful during both of my pregnancies.

Clearly, the claim that technology has usurped women's authority as "knowers" is an overstatement; sometimes it provides information we value deeply. But it's important to remember that more information is not always better. The challenge is figuring out what information will be helpful and what has the potential to undermine. When my doctor pointed to the ultrasound machine and offered, "Let's just look, Annie," it turned out I was looking into Pandora's box, testing my relationship to knowledge. Through the rest of this chapter, I'll offer guidance—from myself as well as from other wise women—about how to navigate this terrain.

Knowledge Before Birth: Preparation

Raquel thought she knew it all going into her first birth. She and her husband were both in their early twenties—excited and, perhaps more to the point, confident about what their delivery would entail. "We were so cocky," she reflected. They hadn't done much reading, and she recounted with a bit of a shudder their experience in birthing class.

> I still remember, my husband—he has this weird sense of humor—they were passing around forceps and he was like, "Can I get a pair of these for salad?"—never dreaming we'd end up using them in a different way . . . And [the instructor was] like, "You need a mantra and you need a focal point," and I'm like, "Okay, my mantra is: epidural." I thought I would get an epidural and never feel another thing. I was so unprepared.

Her birth was nothing like what she'd imagined—Raquel labored for more than two days, never had a fully functioning epidural, and despite her daughter's modest size (just over six pounds), required a big tug with forceps for delivery. Raquel emerged with an appreciable vaginal tear and was happy almost exclusively in the fact that she had "a good outcome baby-wise." For Raquel herself, though, it was "terrifying."

But, Raquel told us, it wasn't that she had an ideal that wasn't met. It was, rather, that she hadn't really thought about birth, hadn't prepared herself for the contingencies, and didn't know enough to understand what was happening in the course of her birth or why. Indeed, most of what made it terrifying, she told us, was her lack of knowledge. For her next birth, Raquel made a promise to herself: "I'm going to be educated this time. Whatever happens, I'm not going to feel like I felt last time. Because not knowing what was going on was one of the worst things."

Part of knowing what is going on relies on good communication between a woman and her doctor or midwife during birth, and I'll get to that later. Part of it, though, relies on knowing a little something about birth beforehand. The trick, of course, is figuring out what information will make the difference.

When Raquel became pregnant again, she picked up *Williams Obstetrics*— a medical tome on the bookshelf of almost every medical student and obstetrician—and read it cover to cover. This time around, she was going to approach birth differently: she wanted to know the medical facts, she wanted to know what the doctors knew (and I'm sure she ended up reading more of that tome than many of my colleagues ever did despite board certifications). It's this sort of information—translated and distilled, perhaps—that the Boston Women's Health Collective wanted to make available with the publication of *Our Bodies, Ourselves* just over forty years ago. That was a time, by all accounts, when most doctors were men and paternalism reigned. The groundbreaking publication was, in the words of one of its original authors, an effort to counter the notion that "women didn't really need to know about their bodies." Now we know we do—but just as *Our Bodies, Ourselves* has swelled from a pamphlet to nearly 1,000 pages, the information available has in effect exploded—and women are faced with the task of figuring out what they need to know and what they can afford to miss.

Mother of two Tonya bumped up against this quandary in her first birth. She hadn't thought much about possible complications because it didn't feel like there was any reason to. She certainly hadn't considered picking up a medical textbook. Pregnancy wasn't a disease, and she felt fine—great, in fact—until an early August evening when everything changed. Just home from work, she was wet—wetter than the usual sneeze made her, and she feared her water had broken. When she looked in the light, she saw that she was standing in a puddle of blood. But it wasn't, according to Tonya, the blood that was so terrifying; it was the *not knowing* what was happening, and why.

It turns out that Tonya had an undetected placenta previa—a condition in which the edge of the placenta is too close to the cervix. Two ultrasounds had missed it, but it made itself known with that evening's terrifying gush. Once she arrived at the emergency room, she was left in a room for thirty minutes before she was seen, then greeted with what felt to her like "mass confusion"— doctors frantically trying to stabilize her, but holding back not just assurances but information. Two days later, the source of the gush was finally disclosed; her baby was delivered by cesarean within the week.

A big part of what she said was bad about her first birth was that she knew nothing about her condition; it had never crossed her mind to read up on placenta previa, much less any of the other complications that could have occurred. And so, she said, the lesson she'd pass on to an expectant mom would be "to take time to educate herself of the possibilities of what could happen, to know the positive outcomes of what could happen along with the negative." In her second birth, she'd read more about complicated pregnancies, and it helped. "I already knew ahead of time during the pregnancy that there was a higher risk involved—pregnancy carries risk anyway—but I had a higher risk because of what had previously happened, and that gave me enough to go on."

It's not that women should (as the unwelcome cookie-wrapped fortune advises) "hope for the best but expect the worst." Far from it. There is plenty of room and reason for thinking positively. But it helps to know in advance— for example—what meconium is if your birth is one of the many where it shows up. Between contractions is hardly the time to get a sense of what it is and how much you need to worry about it.

We heard this a lot from women whose births were complicated or departed in a significant way from the normal vaginal birth that much of the messaging about "bodies working" and pregnancy being a "healthy state" encourages women these days to anticipate. Recall Jill, for instance, who was completely healthy going into pregnancy, but then met with pregnancy-induced liver disease early in the third trimester. Looking back, she advised other women to engage with a range of possibilities before birth.

> You have to at least consider the possibility that you might even have a C-section. They try to prepare you that it's at least a

possibility, but nobody thinks it's going to happen to them. So you need to at least think that it can happen. Not everybody needs to prepare for my kind of experience, but they should remember that pregnancy is not without risk.

But we also heard something similar from women whose births were relatively uncomplicated. They told us that a certain level of preparation provided critical assurance that everything *was* okay—that what they were seeing was not pathological but normal. Despite her husband's protests that birthing classes were a "waste of time," Jackie told me she was grateful for what she learned there. For instance, she was relieved to learn, pre-birth, about vernix—the white substance often found covering the skin of newborns, which we doctors often wipe from their faces en route to their mothers' arms. "I think I would have freaked out," she reflected, "and thought there was something wrong with my baby if I hadn't learned about it in my birthing class." Instead, she could rest assured it was normal—a sign that her child was full-term, complete with a bit of natural lubrication in service of her timely entry.

On the other hand, women also caution about overthinking or overpreparing, especially when it comes to possible complications. Jill admonished that there is a "delicate balance" and that while it's important to consider the range of possibilities, "you can read too much and you sort of overthink the whole thing . . . Knowledge is power, but you also have to let it not psych you out too much."

Obstetricians are commonly criticized for their tendency to think about birth as potentially complicated—for the view that "birth can only be declared normal in retrospect." It is a fair criticism. This perspective inclines us to overuse technology, and not a few in my specialty cite it as a justification for unfortunate restrictions on (or criticisms of women who choose) out-of-hospital birth. On the other hand, to deny that pregnancies get unexpectedly complicated is wishful thinking. And as Tonya, Raquel, and Jill all discovered, getting blindsided when things don't go as planned or hoped for doesn't make for a good birth either.

It's a point sociologist Susan Maushart makes with great fanfare in a chapter of her book *The Mask of Motherhood*, provocatively titled "Laboring Under Delusions." She argues that despite the mountains of information available and widespread access to perinatal education, women emerge from birth "battle-scarred, bewildered, and betrayed." The problem, she argues, is that despite the emphasis on education and childbirth preparation, the truth about childbirth is buried, shrouded in silence.

For one, it hurts more than most of us are led to believe. My friend Michelle tells me that she'll never forget a class she took before the birth of her first child. In an attempt to get the expectant moms used to the idea of staying focused on breathing while they were in pain, all were given a clothespin to clip to their earlobe. Michelle—who labored thirty-six hours and ended up with a cesarean—found the clothespin experience helpful only as an exemplar for how useless the class was for conveying what she was in for. She wanted the facts, and she felt betrayed by the sugarcoating that the emphasis on breathing and backrubs encrusted on her pre-birth understanding of labor pain.

On the other hand, is it really helpful to hear, *à la* Maushart—who compared contractions to "volcanic eruptions"—how birth "really feels"?

In the midst of birth, Maushart had the sense—as did many women in the Good Birth Project—that she was going to die, not because she was, but because this is what normal, unanesthetized birth elicits for many women who experience it. What "saved" her, she said, was an epiphany, a moment of insight that what she was feeling was normal—"Childbirth was torment, not because my mind or body was doing it wrong, but, astoundingly, because I was doing it right." It was something she had to figure out for herself, because nothing she'd read or heard told her anything of the sort. The implication is that what women need is straight talk about birth; they need to know what to expect, *really*. No sugarcoating allowed. Citing as evidence the "emergent literature devoted to unmasking the experience of childbirth," Maushart notes:

> It is possible to convey women's experiences . . . What has formerly gone unspoken is not necessarily unspeakable. Where clinical language has failed, emotive, metaphorical, and ironic language can prove astonishingly evocative. But we need ears to

hear it and a willingness to allow the voices of experience as admissible evidence.

But birthing doesn't feel like dying to everyone. For some lucky women, it's minimally painful; for others still, it's orgasmic. Labor feels different to different women; it can even feel different to the same woman in different births. For instance, mother of two Sally told us that her second labor felt so different from her first that she "couldn't believe it could be the same experience." Both labors were in freestanding birth centers, both were supported, but they felt physically different. Her first labor was classically "excruciating and exhausting," while her second "felt like a different area of my body, like tough menstrual cramps, and they were beautiful."

So how do we know what we need to know? The women of the Good Birth Project tell us that it is about balance. You gather enough information going into birth that you have a sense of what you are experiencing and are not taken unawares, but you don't gather so much that it scares or distracts you, makes you unable to focus on what's good and positive about the process or overly worried that something is going wrong. For some women, that balance might be easy to find. But what if it's not? How do we figure out how to find it?

One of my dearest friends, Helen, is ravenous when it comes to knowledge in general—medical knowledge in particular—so it was no surprise that she picked my brain over the course of both her pregnancies, wanting to get a grasp of all matters gestational.

She is also a brilliant professor and teaches a great course on ethical issues in medicine. One gorgeous fall day, the two of us were walking through campus—Helen was pregnant with her second baby and just beginning to show. We were chatting about potential topics for her upcoming class, and I told her about the challenges that arise when babies are born at what we call "the threshold of viability"—at the edge of when neonatologists can reasonably predict that they'll be able to help a premature baby, that aggressive treatment will save a life, that their tools will do more good than harm. She asked me to visit the class, present a case, and let her students grapple with it.

I did so, and it was a great ninety minutes, in no small part due to Helen's gift for leading discussions of thorny topics. But after the class, I noticed something: Helen started thinking differently about her own body—about whether the mid-pregnancy contractions she'd been experiencing were painless and normal, or harbingers of preterm labor. Visits to her midwife (and calls with me) became more frequent, and it was only with the reassurance of periodic testing that is highly predictive of preterm labor and the passage of time that she could settle back into her pregnancy and get comfortable with what we'd call in obstetrics an "active uterus." Her cervix never opened and she ended up delivering past her due date. But the pregnancy was tough, more than tough. And I always will wonder whether our pedagogical tussle with the ethics of preterm labor was at least in part to blame.

Putting aside what will certainly be an enduring question for me—as girlfriend, confidante, and doctor—I do think there is a broad lesson to be drawn from Helen's experience. That is, there's a certain kind of knowledge that's absolutely key to a good birth: knowledge about yourself. Whether information will be helpful or harmful varies from woman to woman, and a hard look inside can provide a helpful sieve.

So if you are pregnant, it may be helpful to think about childbirth preparation not as a class aimed at competence or mastery of a swath of information, but as a way to engage—before the event—with labor and birth from *your own* perspective, to regard birth from where you are, situated in a pregnant body, on the brink of giving birth. Imagine it as a process of self-discovery, an opportunity to look inside at who you are and what you hope for in the process that lies ahead.

You may be surprised to hear that I attended birth classes and that I think of them as potentially helpful for anyone, whatever their knowledge of anatomy and physiology, of the science or spirituality of birth. There is something to putting yourself there, in the position of someone preparing and looking ahead. I will tell you that it all sounds different from the student side of the room: the signs of labor; the sock stretched over a lightbulb to portray what an infant's head does to the cervix; the process of cesarean, and how long it takes to recover. All take on an air of gravity (if you will) when you are in the birthing body.

That hard look inside is helpful for other reasons as well. In addition to abundant information about anatomy and physiology are the abundance of options for birth. It's hard to pick up a maternity magazine and not read about the pros and cons of various locations, interventions, and types of providers. Women tell us these are important topics to consider as well. But they emphasize the importance not just of knowing what options are out there, but which ones make the most sense for you. As mother of two Maria noted:

> I think it is just really important to be informed. Like I know there is this debate about whether you should have an epidural or you shouldn't, and I don't think there is a right answer, but I just feel it's a decision people need to make based on some knowledge—or experience.

For first-time moms, experience is deeply valuable but largely out of reach—and I'll talk more about that later in the chapter. But if you are one, you can draw on things you know about yourself: how you feel about medical information (does it make you feel worried or empowered?) and hospitals (do they make you feel safe or scared?), how you deal with blood or pain, how you manage uncertainty, how different spaces feel to you.

Through the process of discovery—as you gather knowledge about that interface between you and birth—many birthing classes and books will encourage women to write things down. The implication is that there can be some material evidence of a woman's knowledge about birth and what she wants from the birth experience, that such preparation should culminate in some sort of final report leading into birth, often in the form of a "birth plan," though it can take a variety of forms. But when it comes to the sort of knowledge we really need for birth, how necessary is this writing bit we're all encouraged to do?

I do think that writing what you want or hope for in the course of delivery can be a helpful exercise for some women. For one, it can make you engage with birth, really think about what might be in store, talk through hopes and fears with the people you love, and make sure you've made the best possible choices for yourself. It can be a useful approach to sifting through those mountains of information I talked about earlier. And having something written down is also a helpful way to connect with a doctor or midwife you might not have met before and communicate things that could get lost amid the events and urgencies of birth.

I don't think this sort of advice is specific to birth, though. Indeed, lists can be helpful whenever we enter the doors of a medical facility. I often counsel patients, friends, and family to write down questions and preferences in advance of medical appointments, whether or not they have anything to do with pregnancy. There's so much information (and so little time) that it's good to have a way to gather your thoughts and the pieces of information that seem most important, before you are in the moment. As first-time mom Tess said, "Once you get [to the hospital], you kind of forget everything. You're just kind of in the moment and you don't think about all the things that you've been planning for." It's helpful to have some notes in your pocket to make sure you get your questions answered and points across.

In birth, though, the act of anticipatory writing has morphed over the years into the "birth plan"—a ritual of sorts that many women understand as expected preparation for birth. Gather information about your options, about the hospital or birthing center where you will deliver, about yourself, and distill it into a manifesto of sorts, describing the birth you intend to have. Rule followers like me might think it is something required, something for which a conscientious mom-to-be would carve out time and effort—evidence that we've done our homework. But as the women of the Good Birth Project discovered, the pitfalls of the birth plan, as broadly understood, are several.

For one, birth isn't something you can plan. You can have an idea about how you'd like your birth to go, which may be situated at a distance (or not) from that of your doctor or midwife. But births rarely ever go as planned, and there are always surprises. Both doctors and midwives I interviewed told me they worried most about women who come in with the four-page birth plan, the bulleted list specifying everything from what they want for pain control and how they want it offered, to the song they want playing while their child is crowning. As first-time mom Lynn cautioned:

> Prepare as much as you can, but also understand that when it's actually happening it may be completely different than what you expected and everything that you prepared for. Just be aware of

that and try not to be too rattled. This is just one of those things you can't plan.

First-time mom Corey told us that writing a birth plan had been on her to-do list, but she never managed to get it done, which was fine. "If I'd handed the nurses a birth plan," she reflected, "they probably would have been fine with it, but, to be honest, even by that point it would have been a joke, because everything was already so different that it just didn't matter at all. Would have been a funny thing to read back over, I guess."

As was the case for many first-time moms, for Corey birth was just different from how she'd imagined it. She'd wanted to "avoid medical interventions," but nearly two weeks past her due date, she was more than ready to give birth. "By that point, I was just so ready to have her and not be pregnant anymore that I just didn't care . . . So I let that go very quickly and easily." As her birth unfolded, the birth plan she imagined was jettisoned, by necessity, but in its place was birth itself, and better on many counts.

> I thought I would try to do it without pain medication—you know, my fear is that it would stall labor, or that things would move along more slowly. That didn't seem to be true at all. My fear about the doctor being someone I'd never laid eyes on—he was wonderful, he was super caring and I'm glad it ended up being him. I wanted to be in the tub, but the rocking chair was the most comfortable thing. The environment of the room could have been more homey, but it was just my husband and I, and we kept the lights low.

As Corey discovered, birth can surprise you. It's important not to put too much stock in any one preference. Avoiding intervention sounds good until intervening is safer than not; giving birth in a tub might sound right until you get into the perfect rocking chair. Once in a while, that grumpy male doctor you'd avoided having prenatal appointments with will surprise you— pleasantly—as he helps you usher that baby into the world. *Birth* will surprise you, so a big part of preparation is not about translating what you've learned of birth into specific plans, but about gathering strength and resources for the ride.

This brings me to the sort of preparation I've personally found to be most important to a good birth: being prepared for things to veer from an ideal. As important as it is to think positively, it is also important to be realistic, to engage to some degree with the messy and complicated reality that is giving birth, with information that doesn't fit into idealized plans.

This is no easy task. It was David, my children's pediatrician, who appreciated that I wasn't prepared in this way for William's birth. It takes a special pediatrician to tell a mother of three and obstetrician that she isn't adequately prepared, that she needs to reorient, and in a firm but gentle e-mail David did just that. I'd been back and forth countless times with the surgeon we consulted: I was set on breast-feeding Will immediately after birth; the surgeon was firm that Will eat nothing until we knew what was going on. As we tussled about it, I comforted myself by imagining I could feed William surreptitiously—slip him a sip of fresh colostrum—if I couldn't convince the perinatal team of my view.

About a week before William's birth, with plenty of compassion but in no uncertain terms, David helped me see that once Will was out of my body, whether I fed him or not, we weren't going to go into "normal baby mode": William would be whisked away and spend his first day in the intensive care unit being studied and pricked. It was something I should have known—perhaps did know—but it was a picture that needed to be painted with a firm stroke, an image from which I couldn't turn away. I am grateful to David for not just painting a rosy picture, for not just joining the chorus of voices telling me everything was going to be fine. For I found the shift that conversation engendered to be utterly valuable, an opportunity to assemble the resources I knew I'd need to make my way through. Indeed, knowing that the pediatricians would soon be calling the shots led me to insist on an extended chance to connect with William in the operating room, before our NICU odyssey began.

And so the value of planning for birth, it has always seemed to me, but never more so than now, is best understood as a gathering of resources—information about yourself and your birth—that will most realistically help you shape, navigate, and relish its unfolding.

Knowledge During Birth: Communication

As much as we'd like to get everything settled in advance, much of the time birth entails the unexpected and requires an open heart and mind—and perhaps most of all, open ears. Indeed, women tell us, one of the things most important to a good birth is good communication. They want to know what's happening to their body and their baby, and they want someone who knows how to tell them in a way they understand.

No doubt, with changing shifts and busy wards, communication can suffer—and so can we. Indeed, such was a major source of frustration and offense for Maisie during her first birth experience. "I went to the hospital for a routine sonogram . . . and they said they thought he was only about three pounds, very underweight for thirty-five weeks. So they sent me up to the birthing floor with some paperwork and said, 'Just give these papers to the woman at the desk, then she'll tell you what to do from there.'

"That's all they told me." The conversation in the darkened ultrasound suite didn't leave Maisie with a sense that she was going to give birth that day—far from it. "I thought I was just dropping off papers." She rode the elevator to the labor ward thinking about the bus schedule, which route she'd be taking home, what was in the fridge for dinner.

But once she arrived on the birthing floor, she sensed that something more was planned for her and her baby and that she'd been left out of the loop. Her suspicions were confirmed when a nurse peeked her head through the double doors of Labor and Delivery and offered, "Oh, don't worry, we'll get that peanut out in no time."

Looking back on her first birth, Maisie told us, "I felt so betrayed."

I can imagine why, and it may well be that the doctors who cared for her deserve her disdain. But if you are pregnant or giving birth, there are things you can do to shore up your sense of authority even when information is not as forthcoming as you wish it were. First, remember you can ask. If you don't understand why you are headed up to the birthing floor, why someone is asking you to undress, why they are doing a test or drawing blood, ask. It's your body. You deserve to know. We doctors (and midwives) need to take the time to tell women what we are proposing to do and why, with clarity and compassion.

Second, remember that there are constraints on what information can be disclosed and when. Sometimes the constraint is simply time. One of the things I have found to be most challenging about obstetrics is that it often feels like you should be in two (or more) places at once: in one room talking with someone who has just learned she is miscarrying, and in another room explaining to a woman in Maisie's situation why it might make sense to induce labor early.

Other times, constraints have to do with roles and who should be providing information. Ultrasound technicians are often not allowed to speak with patients, since they won't predictably know the whole situation or the options for treatment, so they can't fill in the gaps. I've come to believe that there are good reasons for tight lips, having caught several friends as they started to plummet toward panic because they'd been given incomplete or inaccurate information.

This is all to say that when information trickles in slowly, try not to feel betrayed—not at first, at least. Sometimes a little silence is better than the enduring din of misinformation, the echo of unfounded worry.

But I urge childbearing women not to go passive either. As Maisie and so many other women tell us, open communication is key to a good birth. If information seems less than forthcoming, ask and press for it. Don't be afraid to get clarity about what's going on, to ask questions of the people taking care of you. There might be time or role-related constraints, or your doctor might need reminding that there is a patient in the body—that you are there and, of all people, you need to know what is going on.

Indeed, good communication can make a world of difference, regardless of how a birth unfolds. Mother of two Cara found this to be true during both her births, which at first blush were very different experiences—an early emergency cesarean and a late VBAC, after which she felt "triumphant." Cara is a fan of the idea of "natural birth," so you might think she'd mourn the first and celebrate the second, but she found the good in both in a shared, if unexpected place.

Just shy of thirty-five weeks pregnant, Cara was the guest of honor at a baby shower at her parents' house in the North Carolina mountains, three hours from the nearest hospital, where she planned to deliver her first baby. She'd recently learned that her baby was in a "transverse" position—side to side, and had begun exploring approaches to coaxing him into the head-down position so she could deliver vaginally. But as she was unwrapping a silver rattle from her mom, her water broke. She called her midwife, who said, "Get [to the hospital], and stand on your head so the [umbilical] cord doesn't prolapse"—the worry being that the cord might slip out the hole in her amniotic sac, through her open cervix, and blood flow to the baby could be cut off. Cara somehow endured the bumpy, upside-down ride to the hospital. Once there, "everything, finally, was calm." An ultrasound showed the baby was fine, though still sideways, and Christopher was born via uncomplicated cesarean forty-five minutes later.

No doubt Cara was disappointed. "I was really hoping for a natural labor," she reflected, "and that was about as unnatural as it gets." But if it wasn't what she had envisioned, what she'd hoped for, she told us, "I was really happy."

Yes, a healthy baby was the big reason. But what also made her happy was the way things happened, the way she was kept abreast of the unanticipated situation by her doula, who met them at the hospital when they finally arrived. The uncertainty she experienced during the ride to the hospital behind her, what made the difference was knowledge that came through good, play-by-play communication during surgery. As she explained:

> The anesthesiologist allowed my doula to come into the delivery room with me, and it turned what could have been a really negative experience for me into a positive one. She could explain everything that was going on—she kept us calm and talked us through everything . . . I am a huge proponent of doulas because of what she did for us with the C-section. Imagine that—we thought she was going to help us with a natural labor, and she helped us have a good C-section.

The right doula can do this beautifully. So can the right doctor or midwife—or anesthesiologist, who through my own cesarean births I've come to appreciate, with our intimate colloquy on the north side of the blue drape. Some of this you can plan, but some is a matter of good fortune and openness to good things where you least expect them, like operating rooms you never thought you'd enter.

The quick-and-dirty version of Cara's second birth is that she got to deliver vaginally, and that was great for her—a corrective to a sense of loss she felt looking back on Christopher's surgical entry into the world. But according to the longer version, the good in her second birth wasn't about just delivery mode. It was, again, about knowledge through good communication.

Having found a group of hospital-based midwives who were eager to help her get her vaginal birth, she carried her second baby past her due date and finally went into labor on a stormy November night. After a long labor and a quick tug with a vacuum, she delivered Layton vaginally—a "triumph" for her. But there was more to it—communication in a moment of uncertainty helped to make her vaginal birth *good* when her baby's heart rate dropped and the midwife had to call in a medical team.

> [My midwife] explained everything to me, which is what I needed. She was looking at me in the eyes, even with that oxygen mask on. She introduced me to everyone who came in the room so I didn't feel invaded, talked me through the pushing and did the suction cup for one push, and he came out . . . The very end was a little bit frightening, but it went so well, I think because she explained everything to me so well, and talked me through it, and I felt like I did it the way that I wanted to do it.

Cara didn't, really, give birth the way she'd hoped or envisioned—standing up, no oxygen mask, no vacuum. But the mid-delivery rapport she shared with her midwife made letting go of that imagined birth and embracing her very own, with its unexpected twists and turns, second nature. She discovered that the good in birth is not about getting exactly what she'd planned, but feeling like she knew what was going on and why. "Afterwards," she puzzled, "my midwife kept coming in and sort of apologizing for using the vacuum and having to put me on the bed and not letting me have the baby standing up." None of that mattered, Cara told us, and she assured her midwife, "No, it was perfect. It was just the way I wanted it."

Indeed, plenty of women in the Good Birth Project told us how good communication made a huge difference for them, though why it mattered varied. For several it was an invaluable deterrent against self-blame; it provided reason—beyond themselves—that their birth went differently from how they'd hoped. It was a way to dispense with mommy guilt and understand birth and bodies as physiologically complicated and, if powerful, also imperfect. Mother of two Shyama told us she was "totally calm and okay" with her cesarean because she'd discussed it at length with her doctor, who "sat down, and talked to me and explained everything that she was doing, my options—things like that. Put me at ease." As a result, she told us:

> It wasn't like someone took away the experience from me, or that
> I was forced to do it. It was more, "Okay, I'm not progressing.
> I've been trying since two in the morning, I'm ten days late, the
> heart rate's dropping." It was more stressful waiting and moni-
> toring than actually going in and having the C-section.

In the end, women tell us that good communication before, during, and after birth is an important part of them understanding their births as "good." As I've said before, it's not something childbearing women can orchestrate, but intuition can take us a good bit of the way. Finding a provider whom you can relate to, whom you "click" with, who takes time to answer your questions, and who seems to care about experience as well as outcome will help ensure a flow of information during birth and in the days that follow.

Of course, we can't always predict how our providers will behave. Mother of two Amity concluded after both her births that "how accessible and participatory your birth team is, is totally key." That ideal wasn't met in her first birth, in which a sudden drop in the fetal heart rate nearly bought her a cesarean.

> I had no idea what was happening—everything was going
> okay and now it's all going to hell in a handbasket and I

don't know why. I felt like, shouldn't I be allowed to participate in at least knowing what's happening to my body and to my baby? In hindsight, I guess when things are really crazy, the doctor's first concern is not explaining everything to you. But at some point that should have happened. And it ruined it for me.

At some point it should have happened. Indeed, the wisdom here is that, even if a conversation can't happen in real time, it need not ruin your birth. It can happen afterward—a good (even competent) practitioner can fill in the blanks, and that's something that women tell us can be immensely satisfying, and empowering as they think about heading toward subsequent births and the inevitable uncertainty they entail. Mom of two Whitney offered that she arranged to talk to her doula postpartum, to "go over the story with her, tell my story, fill in the blanks. It was a really important part of the whole process for me. Really memorable."

Ultimately, it's worth remembering that assessments of birth evolve. First-time mom Lynn had some scary moments in her delivery—not the least of which was when her son was delivered with forceps after she'd pushed for hours. When we asked Lynn for an overall assessment of her birth experience, she replied, "Now? It's really good." But, she cautioned, "it takes a little bit of time for you to look at it that way." The window of knowledge to inform that judgment doesn't just open and close—you can gather information over time to help you make sense of what happened and why, even if wasn't clear immediately after birth. It might happen at a six-week postpartum appointment, or in the park or grocery store if you are one to compare birth stories; it might happen in the pages of this book. Remember, you can ask your doctor to explain what happened and why—when you are ready to hear it, even later on when you are in for an annual visit. The stories of our births evolve over years, and they are worth writing and re-writing, making sense of them through the lenses of information and experience.

Knowledge Through Birth: Experience

I would say I thought I was mentally and physically prepared for [my first baby], but that was a lie—I lied to myself. I just don't think you can prepare for something that you have no experience with. And so, as many books as you read, there's nothing that can prepare you for the first contraction. Nothing.

—SALLY

There is one more piece to the knowledge that makes for a good birth: it is the knowledge of experience, of birthing itself.

If the notion of gathering information before and during birth feels over-whelming, don't let it. For as much as we write and reflect on birth, there is nothing like doing it—nothing really that can prepare you for the experience or provide the wisdom it imparts. It's like skiing (or parenting or sex—or you name it). You can read and think about it all you want, but until you've done it, you can only imagine. You have to point your tips down the hill and give it a go. And I've found this to be as true for so-called experts as it is for anyone. Take, for instance, the respective experiences of Kate and Sidney.

Kate was the first midwife I ever met, the woman my sister-in-law Diane had chosen to attend her first birth. They had clicked right away, and I could see why. She was warm and accessible and exuded a calm confidence that I could only imagine would be just the thing to make impending (and actual) labor seem manageable. And she talked to my brother like he, too, was expect-ing. I'd never seen anything quite like it, and I was intrigued. An obstetrical resident at the time, I'll admit I felt slighted at Diane's decision to eschew the likes of my intended profession, but once I met Kate, I understood the draw.

Kate wasn't against technology. In fact, she allowed the three of us to slip into the medical office where she worked, after hours, so I could take a peek at Mike and Diane's fetus with the ultrasound machine and give my best guess as to gender. What I saw on the screen looked like a girl, but it's always harder to make the call about sex on the absence (rather than presence) of a certain body part. I was much more certain about what I saw in Kate: she exuded the best of midwifery—robustly holistic treatment—and I was moved by it. It made me want to get pregnant; it made me want to know more people like her; it made me want to *be* like her.

Kate did also toe the usual midwifery line, and apparently worked long and hard on Diane to think about laboring without pain medication. She managed to convince my brother (who annoyingly entreated his wife to give it a go), but Diane never wavered from her original stance: "I want drugs," she repeated to anyone who wondered—and she got them, happily, through an epidural catheter placed midway through the good birth of my niece. Diane never looked back.

But Kate did.

When Diane got pregnant again, she called Kate right away, but Kate wasn't practicing anymore. She'd had a baby of her own, was staying home for a while. As is typical of Diane (both a social worker and *People* magazine junkie), she pressed for more of a scoop, and got one: "Labor," Kate told her, "kicked my butt." It made her feel like she'd been lying to people about how labor feels, like she'd been misleading them. As Diane tells it, Kate said labor felt to her like getting "hit in the head repeatedly with a hammer." And the epidural, mercifully, is what finally put an end to that sensation. After she'd experienced it, "Get an epidural, girlfriend" was about the only thing she could imagine telling pregnant women and feeling good about herself. It helped that the tug of full-time mothering was so strong, but giving birth— and having her whole sense of what it was about disrupted—made the decision to take a break from birth attendance that much easier.

Sidney had a different experience entirely. A newly minted obstetrician in a busy private practice, Sidney got pregnant—unexpectedly—with her first child. It was the early 1990s and women were just starting to be a force in the field, though we were still far from the majority. Wanting to prove that she was "tough" and "stoic" and "that [she] could be just as good as those men were and could have a baby too," she didn't take any time off and made every effort to hide her exhaustion.

Near term and feeling beaten by the task of hauling a huge belly up and down the lengthy corridor that was Labor and Delivery, she decided to take the reins—she slipped out of the hospital with a labor-inducing suppository, took a power nap, and put the suppository in place. A few hours passed and she went back to the hospital in labor, and then called her husband, a lawyer who was arguing a trial in a nearby courtroom. "So I induced myself, kind of. Looking back on it, it was the most stupid, ridiculous, unsafe thing to do." At the time, though, it felt like it made sense. "For me personally, it was my baby, my body, and I just needed to get the baby out."

She told us that at first, she felt good about it. She'd delivered her ten-pound baby vaginally, when she wanted to, though she'd torn "from stem to stern" and hemorrhaged to the point that her colleagues and husband were concerned for her life. Her second birth was similarly (if more openly) scripted and fortunately uncomplicated, though she felt like it lacked the intimacy she has learned to cultivate and value in births she has since attended over the years.

Years later, she imagined for us a different scenario—that she'd have let nature take its course, that her first baby would have been so large that a cesarean would have been inevitable, and she wouldn't, after all, have brushed so closely with death that she felt was in some way her "fault." Or perhaps, that she would have connected more with her husband over the birth of their children. "If I had to do it all over again," she reflected, "I would do it differently. I feel badly, really, for my husband. Because the children are our children, but I think he feels like he kind of got cheated . . . I am a little bit sad about my births. I wish they would have been natural."

As happened with Kate, giving birth made Sidney reconsider what she thought birth was all about, though it pressed her in the opposite direction professionally. "For my next life," she told us, "I'm going to be a midwife."

One of the many things remarkable about Sidney and Kate was that both had a wealth of experience and knowledge going into birth. Both had attended hundreds of deliveries. And I can attest that both were and are smart, capable, and incredibly empathic. But neither of them had done it before; what they found was that there was nothing like going through birth to give them a sense of what it entailed, what it was all about, what it meant to them.

There are several things to take away from this pair of stories, and from those of countless other women who would attest that birth is a source of knowledge.

First is just that you can't know everything going into birth, so trying to do so will be an exercise in frustration. The extent to which you misjudge how your birth will be, what exactly you will need, what you find most valuable or memorable or frustrating should not be a metric of how good your birth was—and perhaps more to the point, how well you have navigated the process. It takes going through birth to know these things. As midwife Donna put it, "It's not a test—it's not going to define your whole being if you don't, you know, ace this or something to your expectations. It's just a part of life and you do the best you can."

I agree with Donna that it's not a test, but I'd go further. It's an experience, and going through birth is its own reward. Once you've done it, you've done it. You've given birth. You know something that you could never have known before. And only you can know it.

Second, for many women the knowledge they get through birth shapes how they experience or assess subsequent births and can be immensely valuable. Several women of the Good Birth Project told us how later births got better, how having given birth before gave them a feeling of authority or mastery or calmness. Things that were once surprising or scary or frightening struck them as familiar, imparted an authentic sort of certainty that was formerly missing. They felt wise, experienced—and they valued those feelings; they were part of what made later births good.

For instance, mother of two Eleanor told us her second birth was better because she "knew what was happening in my body." Her water broke at home and she made her way to the hospital, where she settled into a room, received a dose of antibiotics, and waited for labor to begin. If the picture appeared somewhat muddled to those around her (was she in labor yet or not?), she felt sure of herself, sure about what was going on—so sure that she sent her husband away to give a lecture. She explained:

> [Those early contractions] were nothing . . . I told the nurse, "They're nothing compared to what I experienced before." I told my husband, "Go do your work. You have all these deadlines, you're writing a grant, just do it. Just go over there, don't bother me—I'll call you when it's really happening." And then I just knew . . . because I'd gone through it once before.

Natalie also talked about how what she learned and experienced in her first birth allowed her to enjoy her second birth more. But for her it was more a sense of having scratched the itch, having done something she set out to do, having checked a box. Giving birth to Emmie without an epidural freed her up to make a different choice the second time around. In fact, she loved her second birth and told us that the epidural she got that time is a big part of what *made* it good. But, she reflected,

> it's a journey, and who knows . . . If [my second experience] was the first, I might not have appreciated it for what it was. I [look] at it as this really nice, warm, glorious experience, because I had had that first one. So it was all perspective.

It's not that Natalie regretted her decisions or would have done her first birth differently knowing what she does now. "I would not go back and change it," she said, "because it was an experience . . . I know what it's like to have a baby without drugs, and I appreciate that. But I think my second was a kinder labor and delivery."

Raquel also appreciated her most recent birth and felt like she'd finally gotten it right. After three vaginal births, she delivered her fourth by cesarean and told us it was "every bit as positive as any of my other deliveries, if not my best delivery." If she'd hit her stride, though, she didn't wish something else of her previous births. "I wouldn't trade," she insisted. "I mean, how do you say you'd go back and wipe out some of your memories? They are part of what makes you who you are."

Finally, there is a third lesson: knowledge will always elude—in birth, no less than in life. There are things in birth we cannot know. For some it is how a vaginal birth feels, whether you would have lived had you given birth a hundred years ago, how your dad would have reacted had he lived to see you become a mother, what it would have been like to give birth at home, who this child would have been had you made love an hour before or after. Uncertainty is a part of birth: a good birth can be found in accepting that no matter how much we read or how many children we bring into the world, there will always be things we cannot know.

This has been the lesson, for me, of William's birth: what I've come to call the lesson of the ellipse.

As I write, William is just one. He never had that surgery that was threatened on his first day of life. As months passed and he thrived, the urgency to remove the ellipse faded, and we all (surgeons, pediatricians, and parents) settled into a watchful waiting approach, the question being not about whether to operate, but whether to keep looking for something I wish we'd never seen.

When I look at his unscarred belly, I often find myself shuddering, imagining that we were a breath, a word away from the surgeons putting their knife into it. Then I bury my face in his sweet skin, awash with gratitude for the strength we found to say no at the moment we had to say it. William continues to thrive, and we have all but stopped imaging his internal birthmark; it has almost faded from imagination.

I recognize that I may have felt gratitude for a scar had we made a different choice, viewing the deft removal of the offending lesion as a saving grace, worth the brush with risk and inevitable harm that a knife in a newborn belly entails.

And the ellipse is still there, I am quite sure, enduring as birthmarks tend to be. In my continued efforts to press thoughts of it away, I've come to regard it not just as Will's internal birthmark, but as a marker of sorts of the uncertainty that is a part of every birth, every life.

Like the ellipse, uncertainty in birth is something we all understandably try to stare down, capture on film or with a firm diagnosis, conquer with knowledge or intervention or assurance. But there comes a moment when we just have to accept that there are things we cannot know. Like the ellipse that remains literally under Will's skin (and symbolically under mine), uncertainty will accompany us as we embark on the journey of parenthood, as we march forward on the journey of life. It is something we must learn to live with, work around, or make our peace with.

It is both a lesson for birth and birth's lesson for life.

seven

Looking Forward, Looking Back: Birth as Transformation

Whether figured as a death or heroic rebirth, childbirth is ... always a turning-point, a narrative crisis that destroys, confirms or creates a woman's sense of identity.

—TESS COSSLETT

I have been asked if I had the choice again, would I have a child? This is an absurd question. I am not the same person I was before I had a child. That young woman would not understand me.

—SUSAN GRIFFIN

The heart of this book has portrayed women's wisdom about what makes the experience of birth good in real time—the sorts of things that make navigating the white water of parturition both manageable and meaningful: agency, personal security, connectedness, respect, and knowledge. Part of what I've aimed to do is to dismantle the frames that currently dominate the birth debates, and thereby provide women with a better way to parse the options, information, opportunities, and challenges they'll face during pregnancy and delivery.

But for most of our lives, birth is something to be understood in retrospect—something looked back upon, made sense of, or held dear—and from our vantage point as women who have given birth, as mothers. Thus a good birth also has very much to do with what birthing leaves us now that we are on the other side of that channel crossing.

The apt metaphor notwithstanding, birth is not just a passage but a transformation. "You think marriage is something," my mom (married to my dad for thirty-five years) said to me before Grant was born. "Just wait until they put that baby in your arms." I have taken from that gentle admonition two things: one, that with a baby comes breathtaking responsibility; and two, that giving birth entails not just a shift in what you must or should do but in who you are and how the world looks to you.

This is hopeful news—hopeful for the Good Birth Project, and hopeful for women and birth. The good birth is not as subject as one might think to the whims of physiology or fate. It is not just a fact of the matter (it was, or it wasn't a good birth, period) but something that can be understood over time. The good birth is an assessment that can shift according to how we look at our births and their aftermaths, what we come to see as valuable, and who we have become as a result of going through the experience. As such, the process of looking back on birth is as important as the process of looking forward. I take as strong evidence of this the enthusiasm (and deluge) with which we were met when recruiting women for the Good Birth Project, as well as the steady flow of stories that came to me outside the project and which I wove into this book between and among the project's threads. Birth stories have a life to them—they are told and retold, a continued source of meaning across our lives.

This final chapter will entail a shift of vantage point. With a new conception of the good birth in hand, Chapter 7 looks back instead of forward, suggests what women's wisdom can tell you about understanding birth and about understanding yourself now that you have crossed birth's threshold.

If you are pregnant for the first time, this is a chapter you may want to save for when your baby is in arms. Perhaps tuck the book away amid the objects (if there are any yet) you've assembled for your baby's arrival: the snap-clad tees that defy imagination as something to slip over a tiny body, the bassinet in which you will place a swaddled infant who is *yours*, the cloth with which you will perhaps reattach this child to yourself so you can take a walk, fix dinner, or shop (or just hide a bulge). And once you are there, when you are a mother, you can look back, find the positive and profound, think through the many ways in which it was and will be a good birth.

There is no question that the births recounted in this book are different from your own, or from those you have in some way been a part of. No two births are the same. The reasons they are good differ, if sometimes just by a whisper. Just as I've found resonance across women's stories, my hope is that what has emerged through my considering them together will have resonance for you too.

The first and perhaps most important thing I'll tell you is to trust yourself. Do not just dispense with your sense of your birth. I've seen far too many women moved to do so—women who felt good about their births until they felt the tug of the birth wars. If it weren't for my mom and her soup tureen, I surely would have suffered their pull for longer.

Birth war noise was something my neighbor Nancy had to resist after giving birth to her first, more than a decade ago. Nancy is a mother of teenage boys, an editor and writer, someone upon whom I frequently project my future self. When she reflected on her first birth, she focused in particular on the doubt that characterized its aftermath.

Nancy explained that she and her husband had signed up for the local Bradley class and that she loved it for the way it made her feel a part of a birthing community, like she had a collection of confidants and friends with whom to share experience. But near term, her baby was in a transverse position, side to side, and wouldn't budge—an impossible situation for vaginal birth. So she shelved many of the tools she'd collected in birthing class and underwent cesarean, though still with a supportive partner by her side, in the spirit of Bradley's teaching. She found Jeremy's birth immensely satisfying and felt nothing but fondness for the event until she reconnected with her Bradley friends, who started treating her as if she'd suffered an immense loss. "They kept asking me whether I was okay," she told me. "And I was—I was great, ecstatic. But hanging out with them made me feel like I shouldn't be."

Some researchers would ascribe Nancy's elation and acceptance followed by disappointment to the "halo effect," which birth researcher Penny Simkin explains is "frequently observed when a successful and significant event takes place; even though negative undertones or some disappointments are associated with it, these are temporarily overshadowed by the excitement and joy of the moment."

But I would offer that the excitement and joy are *not* muddling, but are the stuff of a good birth—are something to which we should hold fast—and that the disappointment that erupts for some women is a product of the conversations that happen after birth rather than the circumstances or experiences of birth itself. I believe the regret so many women beat back reflects not some deep "truth" made visible by lifting euphoria's haze but a new sense of our birth negotiated in the context of a dialogue that values either normalcy or health above all and that often fails to capture what women value most.

No doubt there is a role for looking at birth with a critical eye, for finding things that you wish had gone differently and considering them as you approach future births or other of life's thresholds. I'm not saying you should just turn away from disappointment felt either in the moment or in birth's aftermath. But it's important to remember that value can be found in contexts other than the birth wars' extremes, in a conception of the good birth that captures what is centrally at issue in it for you.

In debates about birth we have fought so fiercely that we've developed a sort of blindness to birth itself and its central actor. It is not epidurals or spaces or modes of delivery, incisions across bellies or vaginas, gadgets for listening or looking or monitoring. It is birthing that is the important thing—and the life that it punctuates as well as the life it ushers in. What makes birth manageable and meaningful—indeed, what makes it good—will relate in a substantial way to the person or people who have experienced it. A good birth has very much to do with the lives that precede it and the lives that follow.

Before I close, I want to reflect on what women value about birth's aftermath—three ways they tell us birth can transform. I bring these up not as particular aspirations but as examples of the way that birth endures, the way it is an ongoing process, how the good in and of birth is something we can come to understand and embrace over time.

Empowerment

Many women will describe how they felt empowered by birth. Birth can change a woman's sense of her capacity to do things, to act and accomplish things in life. Describing a recent birth she attended, midwife Donna noted:

> That woman's been changed for life. What she can do, and everything. Totally just changed . . . I just can't help but think that a good birth like that really does color your life from then on in. It certainly has colored mine, because I had great births, where people let me do my thing—you know, just really empowered me.

The idea that birth can do this for some women is certainly remarkable. It turns women like Donna into self-proclaimed "birth junkies." It gives others the feeling that they can "do anything"—like mother of three Carmen, who found birth to be "a very empowering experience. And I don't want to use that word as a cliché—I really mean it was empowering. It gave me a whole new sense of being."

The potential for empowerment is part of what is behind some of the most innovative and exciting developments in our field. Take, for instance, the Developing Families Center (DFC), which houses a freestanding birth center in the heart of one of Washington, D.C.'s toughest neighborhoods. It was founded by MacArthur "genius" award winner, octogenarian, visionary, and midwife Ruth Lubic more than a decade ago. While it can boast of far lower rates of premature birth and cesarean delivery among its clients, it also aims to help women achieve a sense of "empowerment" through their birthing experience.

When we visited the DFC, we spoke to several women who had received their care there. They are given the option of delivering either in the local hospital or in the facility itself, and twenty-five-year-old Malia chose the latter option for her second birth. Comparing her experience delivering in the birth center with her prior hospital birth, she told us:

It was just so hugely different in sort of a life-changing way. I mean, I don't really know how to articulate it, but it was—it changed something about me, and I have no idea how to articulate it other than to just say it—it was life-altering.

Now, you might not be surprised to hear that Malia's birth was of the sort often fetishized, as was Carmen's; they were low-intervention vaginal births, followed by post-delivery euphoria. Donna's patient, too, labored quickly, gave birth without anesthesia, pulled the child from her body with her own hands.

"Isn't that just endorphins?" Kim asked me when I described the phenomenon. He was referring to substances the body releases in response to exercise, excitement, love, orgasm, spicy food, and—yes—pain. Nobody denies that endorphins are at play in birth. Many advocates of midwifery care cite endorphin release as a valuable end in birth, as a *reason* even to delay or avoid epidural use altogether. As my weathered running shoes suggest, I can be an endorphin junkie, but I find the press for such in birth a little strange. Just because something results in the helpful release of a particular neurotransmitter, it doesn't mean that it is an end worthy of pursuit. Indeed, there are things that we think entirely optional and maybe a little crazy (ultramarathons, for example) or pathological (bulimia) in which endorphin release has a central role.

Of course, the actual endorphin rush is fleeting—and just part of what sets the stage for post-birth empowerment. But I'd offer that while endorphins can powerfully shore up the foundation for enduring empowerment, there are other ways to get there. Feelings of empowerment need not turn on the vicissitudes of birth and our needs and preferences in the process, of the secretions of our glands, of our bodily experiences in birth's immediate aftermath. Power—even power in and through birth—has many sources.

Empowerment can come from recognizing that the body you live in can do something quite extraordinary in gestating another human being. It can come from holding together as you are pushed to an edge; it can grow out of the intensity of emotion—the elation or sadness or love—you feel in the process or the days that follow.

It helps to remember that power itself is a tricky notion. In 2001, journalist Margaret Talbot parsed power elegantly in a memorable piece in *The New York Times Magazine*. Power, she observed, is usually thought of as the stuff of "female CEOs . . . and Hollywood mogulettes." But there is another sort of power she said interested her and which that issue of the magazine was meant to portray—power that is "complicated, quotidian, intimate, ambiguous."

If our culture thinks about power too narrowly, power in birth has also been pigeonholed. The woman who comes to my office with a stack of articles and requests an early epidural, citing data that it is safe and does not increase the chances of a cesarean, is—according to the dominant narrative—not empowered but somehow "wimpy." I'd counter that this is far from the case. She is at least as empowered as the woman who eschews technology. There are many ways that birth and power are linked, and we should acknowledge and embrace them in their breadth.

As a doctor, I have been moved by power I've seen women exude in the face of loss—the courage they've shown in pushing a baby from their body who will be sick or may even die. This is a sort of power I find unimaginable, but it is there, buried sometimes amid the challenges of the day and untold stories. Remember Katha from Chapter 4, who faced the formidable uncertainty in birth of having a child with a severe heart defect. She might not offer empowerment as one of birth's remnants. In fact, she told us, "It wasn't really about me at all."

But listening to Katha, it's pretty clear that she gained strength through the process. She just doesn't use the same words as Malia or Donna. She doesn't call it empowerment, but it sounds like something similar.

> Well, a week after my C-section, I showed [my husband] that I could do jumping jacks. Like, I think it reinforced the fact that I'm tough and that I can get through things. You know, the first three days were really, really hard, but then it just kept getting better and better, and I kept pushing myself. It made me realize that I'm tough.

It's not that I would advise jumping jacks one week post-surgery (indeed, we encourage women to take it easy for at least six). Rather, this is all to say that there are many ways to derive power through birth, and different women will find power in different ways. If we celebrate some (like enduring the pain of labor), it's worth paying attention to the other places empowerment can be found.

Indeed, it reminds me of a point made by Talbot: that "you see women who occupy positions of power without declaiming they do, women who are too busy living their full and contradictory crazy-quilt lives to think much about being Powerful Women." But in the moments that you have to consider the notion of power, my hope is that your recollections of birth shore up your power rather than call it into question.

Once into the Good Birth Project, mothers started looking different to me. They still do. With babies strapped on or toddlers in tow (or children in college or grandchildren underfoot), they are—among many other things—people who have given birth. And to that end they are powerful, at the very least because of what it demands of a person—any person—to do such a thing. I have come to appreciate that empowerment is abundant, fills the crevices between if not the big rocks that make up experiences of and reflections on birth. To this end, each and every mother is in fact a Powerful Woman—for what she accomplished, insisted on, or just endured in making it across the channel, and then regarding the passage.

Finally, I think it reasonable to reject the quest for empowerment through birth in any of the ways I've offered. You just might be one of those people who don't want or need empowerment through birth, and that's fine. Tonya told us, "I've always been pretty much confident in myself. I've had plenty of experiences that I've had to be strong for in the past, so [birth] didn't really bring up any of those feelings for me."

Wholeness

Birth is not just about power. It is also about relatedness and, perhaps more to the point, integrity, wholeness. The satisfaction I derive from having William in arms, his birth behind us, is not just a measure of having powered through a challenge, but is in feeling accompanied; I have mentioned that giving birth has been a way I've beat back existential loneliness. Birth can be a gift that way.

In approaching William's birth, I remember thinking how nice it was to carry a baby inside my belly, to have both hands free to write and drive and dress myself, to help my boys find a missing Lego piece, to be singular in my focus on work or just making a cup of coffee. I remember one night in particular, propped in my bed, reading a book. My three boys were at last asleep; Kim was downstairs jogging on the treadmill; and there I was, accompanied by the rhythms of my nearly grown fetus doing his dance beneath my skin. Having given birth three times before, I knew too well how birth obliterates that particular sense of intactness, of physical (and perhaps spiritual) integrity. Whether vaginally or through a surgeon's incision, our bodies are transgressed by the birth of our children, they become soft and leaky and shared—and what emerges is a new sort of wholeness that demands keeping track of, tending to, negotiating the space that exists between our children and ourselves.

I am not just talking about order and chaos. I am, rather, talking about how we see ourselves as we march through life, as separate or separable from others. In advising first-time moms on the brink of birth, like most in my field I'd remind them of the signs of labor and reasons to call or come to Labor and Delivery. But I also have offered the suggestion—with an emphatic prod—that they go out on a date, see a movie, or go for a long walk. Because once that baby comes, they will never be able to do it without a bit of divided attention, even if their child is with a trusted babysitter. If we ever thought we were independent of other humans, birth and motherhood reminds us that we are not.

A growing body of evidence shows that fetal cells migrate to mothers' brains and endure there for years. Some mothers find their presence to be physical evidence of our ongoing connectedness, how it is that the pain our children endure could feel like our own, and why maternal guilt is so very powerful even when harm is unavoidable. I wonder sometimes myself whether they've done more for me than put me on high alert for pain or harm— whether they are in fact a source of completeness, helping me dispense with the feelings of fragmentation that characterized my twenties and went by the wayside with the birth of my first child.

Birth connects us to others besides children, however. Indeed, many of the providers we interviewed told us how giving birth helped them understand in a very deep way what their patients were experiencing in birth. Such was the case for midwife Tess, who had been counting on a dose of empowerment through birth. She'd just finished midwifery school and seen her share of "transforming" natural births in line with the mantra that bodies work and drug-free birth was the way to go. From her vantage point as a freshly minted midwife, birth looked "not easy, but like people do it very well."

"But then," Tess told us, "labor hit me like a ton of bricks." It wasn't empowering. It was excruciating, long and painful. There was no endorphin rush, no euphoria. "My birth," Tess reflected, was "hard and awful and it was torture. I mean, really, I think it was torture." Nevertheless, Tess insisted that "the experience was great."

As she talked more, I started to understand. Birth might not have left her feeling any more empowered, but she did find something precious in the remains of that day. "God forbid I had a totally easy first birth," she mused. "I don't know that I would be the midwife I am." It wasn't that she felt like she could climb a mountain now. Rather, she believed that she could understand how her patients felt when the mountain really was too steep. That first birth was good, she told us, because it left her with something that was equally valuable. It left her with *empathy*. She went on to say:

> I'm not the kind of person who is as empathetic as probably other people in my profession. I really need the slap-me-in-the-face kind of experience. Having that experience helped me a lot. It helped me talk to women, helped me empathize. Helped me appreciate the variety of reactions to and feelings about what happens to them, and all the things you go through when you are pregnant.

No doubt birth can impart a new way of relating to others. It is not just about midwives' or doctors' ability to empathize with their patients, though I think it is helpful that way. It is not just about moms' ability to connect with their children, to know what they need and how to protect them. It is, rather, that birth can transform our sense of independence and reliance.

Perhaps this is more a product of parenthood than birthing, of love for

our children, whatever their pathway to our hearts. But birth can be the ful-
crum in the shift, for it does not just bring up these glaring facts of vulnerability, but in bringing them close it also provides a chance to renegotiate, or
just settle into the fact of mortality and the temporariness of life. In its slippery uncertainty, the elusiveness of control, it presses us not just to mourn
life's edges but celebrate what's in between.

For our tenth wedding anniversary, Kim and I splurged on a gift for each
other: a portrait of our family painted by one of our favorite local artists. Her
style is fairly abstract and a touch whimsical. Though she is well regarded in
the art community, we chose her because there is something about the way
people, places, and meaning come through her canvases that has always
stopped us in our tracks.

Getting painted by Jane gave us a glimpse of why. Before she took up
the paintbrush for the commission, she came over to our house, spoke to
us, and played with the boys. While we enjoyed her company, she must
have watched us and gotten a sense not just of what we looked like but of how
we related to one another and the world around us. For we felt not just depicted, but revealed by the piece we picked up at her gallery three months
later.

In it, she painted the three boys we had at the time doing what they usually
do—one was on Kim's shoulders, another had a toy truck in hand, and a third
gleefully headed down our jungle gym's slide. My mom was seated in the
background sipping something out of a mug (strong coffee, to be sure), wav-
ing to the children. Everybody looked pretty relaxed, with the possible exception of me, standing with arms outstretched, at the worried ready to catch a
boy who would inevitably tumble in his enthusiasm on our backyard bricks.

When Will arrived two years later, we asked her, with some trepidation, to add him to the portrait, and she immediately agreed. Again she visited and met Will; she took the canvas home, and weeks later returned with
what struck a few of us that knew it well as an entirely new piece. The
new brushstrokes were few—just Will now perched in the crook of my
arm. I don't think she changed my countenance, but it seemed wholly different. No longer at worried ready, with Will in arms I had finally settled in.

Women like me, in their forties with children, will tell you that news of a
pregnancy is more often greeted with a response like "Why?" or "Really?"

than the usual "Congratulations." Indeed, one of my best friends from college asked me both lovingly and skeptically, "Are you crazy?" when I told her of Will's impending arrival.

Other women, though, seem to understand more clearly the promise of birth. If for many it's about that seat at the table, the process brings something more—something that settles us, gives us something other than power, something more akin to peace.

Wisdom

This brings me to a third sort of transformation. Birth is a source of knowledge. And a good birth is one that makes us wiser. Birth has changed the way I think about love and loss, safety and risk, connectedness and loneliness. I know what it is like to gestate a child, to experience the simultaneous occurrence of intense new love and separation. To understand that love demands not just affection and attraction, but space between. These things have made me value my births not for how they happened but for what they have left me.

Indeed, this is why I looked to women themselves to craft a notion of a good birth. The experience of giving birth changes us; it changes what we value in birth and in life. It teaches us about ambivalence and uncertainty. It is a lesson in control and its limits. If we strive to be agents of our births, we come to recognize that something profound is happening to us—something we cannot orchestrate. If we strive to feel safe and secure in the context of birth, we come to recognize that risk is unavoidable in birth no less than in life. If we strive to feel connected in birth, we come to realize that birth is both a pulling apart and coming together, a challenge to the notion of an independent self. If we strive to become wiser through birth, we come to recognize that there will always be things we cannot know.

Finally, remember that birth is a beginning—of the life of your child, of your life as a mother, of living in and negotiating that new shared space. There are ways in which your good birth is still in process. So you best turn back around and look ahead to watch, experience, and relish its unfolding.

Common Ground: Notes to Maternity Care Providers

I still believe that everybody deserves a midwife and not everybody needs a doctor.

—STELLA, OBSTETRICIAN

I don't want to bad-mouth technology—it's wonderful when you need it.

—DONNA, MIDWIFE

Undoubtedly women have plenty to teach one another about what makes for a good birth, about how to find the positive and profound in their childbirth experience. But as I distilled their wisdom and my own reflections into practical advice for mothers and mothers-to-be, it struck me that they had a steep mountain to climb, in no small part because of how we talk and think about birth and how we care for women doing it.

When I say *we*, I refer not just to doctors, but to midwives and nurses and doulas and others who attend women giving birth. I refer not just to those who support women laboring, who help them over birth's threshold, but to those who make decisions that shape the way maternity care is provided. I also refer to advocates, journalists, and academics who, with powerful words and stories, illuminate pathways for birth but emphasize resistance and conflict, reinforce the stark and unbending terms of the debate, and beat the flames of the birth wars. We all have a hand in the challenges women face in getting to the good in birth.

Women shouldn't face these challenges alone. There are things that health care providers, advocates, and policy makers can and should do in service of the good birth; wise women can show us the way. Indeed, the women of the Good Birth Project have important lessons to teach us.

In the bickering that is the birth wars, women lose. I have had it with war. I have four boys, and as much as I've tried to expunge from their experiences narratives of violence and conflict, they know about war, put Nerf guns on the top of their Christmas lists every year despite the fact that they never find them beneath our tree, and line up their Lego Stormtroopers in formation. My oldest gravitates toward books about war; he picked up my alumni magazine that showcased Dartmouth's war heroes and read it cover to cover at the kitchen table, in an act of what I could only understand as defiance.

So you might wonder why I use the term *war* to describe the lively and sometimes contentious debates that have characterized the dialogue between obstetrics and midwifery communities for the past several decades. The reason is this: I believe in my heart that there are no winners in war, and this is true of our current dialogue about birth. Obstetric medicine's defenders hurl provocative insults, as in one prominent blogger's claim that "home birth kills," while midwifery's defenders shoot back, implying a "thinking woman" would choose home birth. If I were to step into the fray, I'd add at the very least that the shrillest among them are not providers of maternity care and too rarely if ever evoke robust data about what the experience of birthing means to women themselves.

I can tell you that the birth wars have had an effect, though perhaps not the one advocates may have hoped for. They have set the stage for guilt and self-doubt among childbearing women who face stark and false choices among caricatured versions of birth rather than the authentic and messy and uncertain options that birthing, wherever you do it, entails. I weave this collateral damage throughout the book, most notably in the Introduction and in Chapter 5, but the material I have in my database could fill a tome.

The birth wars also set the stage for feelings of abandonment and isolation. A double-digit percentage of women who opt for out-of-hospital birth will end up being transferred to a hospital for delivery; among women who need or want to deliver in hospitals, midwifery care could and should play a central role (more on this below). The bright line drawn between midwifery and obstetrics is often crossed by necessity or need by birthing women—crossing it should not entail a crisis, nor should it engender worries of abandonment or harm. If some midwives view doctors as adversaries, and vice versa, the women under their care would be better served if they viewed them as partners and individuals invested in their patients' well-being. Birthing in the absence of trust can make a woman feel vulnerable and frighteningly alone. Our lack of interprofessional trust has no place at the bedside.

So the first lesson I'd offer is that we should end our bickering, call a truce, and end the birth wars. I like to think that we could step off the battlefield, though there are those who will always be drawn to fight. I will say, though, that the doctors and midwives I interviewed for the project don't see birth options so starkly. They understand, like midwife Donna whose words opened this chapter, that technology is "wonderful when you need it" and that a home or a birth center may not be the right place for a woman to give birth, for a variety of reasons—some medical, some personal, all reasonable and respectable. Like obstetrician Stella whose words also became an epigraph of this chapter, they appreciate the wisdom of midwifery—and that all women, whether they give birth in hospitals or homes, whether their births are "normal" or complicated, need and value the sort of respectful, supportive, and holistic care championed by midwifery's advocates.

Some would say a truce on some fronts has been called. There are efforts to join forces, to bring together the strengths of midwifery and obstetrics, to acknowledge and work toward capturing the ways they complement each other. Midwives now teach students and residents in our medical schools about uncomplicated births, about being with birthing women, in a more thoroughgoing way than I ever observed or experienced during my years in obstetric training. Representatives from the respective organizations have come together on several issues. Making the synergies between midwifery and obstetrics even more robust and visible would go a long way in helping women understand and access choices that make the most sense to them in the context of their own lives—indeed, in pursuing *their own* good births, wherever and however they'd like them to occur. I would urge both sides to continue these efforts, to seek and acknowledge common ground, and let women know when you've found it.

Every woman does deserve a midwife. I agree with Stella—again, one of the obstetricians we interviewed who made this point—but I should explain more of what she means. Stella was once a midwife, and most of us who know her say she still is. She also makes no apologies for technology and is handy with the scalpel when it is required. What she will tell you, though, is, whatever the level of technology or intervention required, women need and deserve the sort of care that midwifery tends to champion: care that is respectful of the woman, baby, and the event of birth as one imbued with meaning; that allows for intimacy and connectedness between the woman and her provider and fosters engagement of family members; and, perhaps most important, recognizes the woman as the central actor in birth's unfolding.

There are three ways to make sure that every woman gets a midwife. The first is to make sure that midwives are available to women wherever they give birth, whatever their resources; we should look to models (like some in Europe) in which midwives hold the central role in the administration of maternity care. Second, we should work toward practices and policies that support a range of safe options for childbearing women, including out-of-hospital birth in experienced hands. Third—and perhaps most controversial—we should examine the disconnect between midwives' eschewing technological intervention and the tenets of respect and empowerment of women that midwifery holds dear. Indeed, as the Good Birth Project makes clear, a woman-centered birth and intervention, even elective intervention, can go hand in hand.

My view is that all of us who attend women in birth need to be midwives of sorts—if we can construe midwifery without the deep skepticism of technology that some of its versions entail. Stella recounted a recent conversation she had with medical students—on their first day of medical school—that makes the point.

A medical student asked Stella, "Isn't it true that a midwife provides a patient-centered birth and a physician provides a doctor-centered birth?"

Stella replied, "You are going to be a physician. You had better be patient-centered from this point forward. That is what we expect of every one of you."

If patient-centeredness defines midwifery, then no doubt any of us who attends birth—whatever our degree or relationship to technology—should be a midwife. We all need to recognize the childbearing woman as the central actor in the unfolding drama that is birth, whatever the circumstances of her birth—whether she wants to give birth in a tub at home or with an epi-dural at a hospital, whether pregnancy and birth are accurately construed for her as "healthy" or whether they threaten her life due to known or unforeseen complications. "I hope that I could be considered a midwife for those high-risk deliveries," said Stella, whose practice is full of women with complicated, sometimes life-threatening pregnancies, "that the patient would have the same sort of experience in terms of relationship, and as patient-centered as we can make it." I hope that we all could. It is, to my mind, among the worthiest of goals.

Remember, you can't control birth. Women know it. So do we, deep down. But all of us try to, one way or another. We parse it up into stages, name them, describe for each other what they mean. We doctors in particular expect one another and ourselves to keep close tabs, weigh and measure, monitor laboring women with ever more sophisticated technologies, find ways to test and sometimes treat, shove risk to the side and work toward its elimination, riveted by the dangers of birth and the task of keeping them at bay. Others insist on birth's safety and normalcy, on the functionality of the body, on the view that it was "designed" for the work of parturition; though it looks different from constant monitoring and managing of delivery and birth, this tendency has just as much to do with control. Both are efforts to manage the uncertainty that goes along with birth.

When a patient's wishes, or another health care provider's approach to birth, threatens your feelings of control, think before you push back. The heart of the conflict is not ultimately about who is "in control" of birth, for nobody really is. So if your patient refuses an intravenous line, think before you insist on placing it; for both of you, its presence or absence in her arm is probably less about its potential to avert or cause morbidity, and more about access to the body, about penetrability. Conversely, if your patient is drawn toward technology, finds comfort and even empowerment in it, listen to her—consider the ways in which her view is absolutely reasonable. And the little things can make a big difference. If a woman is undergoing cesarean, bring the baby to her cheek, let *her* decide when she feels ready to have the pediatrics team take the child to the nursery. If a woman wants to wear her own clothes rather than a hospital gown, why not? Let go where you can; it will help you help your patient get the sort of control women say is critical to a good birth.

Risk is in the eye of the beholder. In a letter to *The New York Times*, Katharine Wenstrom, a maternal-fetal specialist at Brown University, offered, "If you knew that your birthing experience was going to be completely normal from start to finish, arranging a home birth would make sense. But no woman knows that." She is right. No woman knows that her birth will be normal start to finish, free of risk or harm. But the fact is that though we doctors can keep certain risks at bay in hospitals, our instruments and approaches do not banish risk as completely as we might imagine.

There is no way to eliminate risk in birth. If you are a doctor, you might think of certain risks as eliminable and thus somehow taboo (like the newborn in intensive care because of a delayed cesarean—that home birth that could have ended differently) and others as unfortunate but part and parcel of responsible obstetrical care (like a uterine incision that graces a baby's face during a cesarean, an indicated, perhaps lifesaving intervention). Others might recognize and more readily condemn harm that results from obstetric interventions—perhaps view it as an unnecessary by-product of the medicalization of birth in the United States. Indeed, anthropologist and obstetrician Claire Wendland observed that most obstetrical studies fail to consider a cesarean incision as injurious. If a woman's cervix is lacerated, if she develops a vaginal hematoma, if her newborn's clavicle gets broken—these are risks considered in the balance. "But the intentional wound," Wendland offers, "is exempt by fiat." Because we doctors intend it, we don't see it as an injury.

One of the things that surprised me was that many women chose out-of-hospital birth not because it gave them access to a peak experience, but because, to them, it felt safer. Mother of two Molly, who lost a set of twins and then had what she described as a traumatic cesarean, decided for her third delivery to give birth at home. She told us that "the biggest reason" she chose home birth was because of "the safety," citing a paradox of which we all should take note: "They tell us during the whole pregnancy, 'Don't take drugs—it's not good for the baby,' and yet the moment you step into a hospital they are pushing drugs on you!" If we are committed to facilitating the best obstetrical outcomes for women, we need to figure out why hospitals feel so very threatening to women, figure out ways to make the hospital a place that feels less scary and more reassuring, especially to women who are likely to benefit from technology's ready access.

The other thing to know is that for women giving birth, part of the safety that matters has to do with the experience in real time. Brushes with danger, whatever their result, endure for women; they are among the things that birth leaves them. Feeling safe in birth is not just a means to an end—a means to a faster or less painful labor. Rather, it is an end in itself: part of a good birth. We will never settle the question of what a safe birth is unless we recognize that risk is in the eye of the beholder, and safety must always be in part a measure of how the women we care for understand it.

There is more to a good birth than meeting expectations. We all have been fed a line that expectations are key to a good birth. So many of the providers I interviewed said they thought so—like Sidney, who told us that the most important thing was to "listen to the patient and . . . understand their expectations," or Scott, who thought the root of women's disaffection with birth was their higher-than-reasonable expectations. Studies have tried to describe the relationship between satisfaction and expectations in birth. If there is one, it is complex: taken together the data suggest that women whose births exceed their expectations or meet high expectations are more satisfied; women who have low expectations are less satisfied. If these data are right, one might conclude that in birth what matters is the expectations themselves rather than whether we meet them or not. Low expectations promise disappointment. We *want* our patients to expect a good birth, and we need to know how to do our part in making that happen.

It's not about being able to meet a litany of requests outlined in a lengthy birth plan, or happening to attend a woman who is blessed with a generous pelvis or a quick labor: such would be a tall order, often realistically out of reach. But not to worry. What I found in the Good Birth Project is the mismatch between concrete expectations (like getting an epidural, or getting in the tub) and outcome doesn't predict a good birth at all. Rather a good birth had much more to do with meeting a woman's emotional needs—needs I outline in the book. Many of the women I interviewed had births that strayed considerably from what they had hoped for or expected. But what determined whether their birth was good had more to do with their feelings of agency, security, connectedness, respect, and knowledge than whether their births unfolded according to plan. The bottom line is that a good birth is within reach, however it unfolds physiologically, and as maternity care providers we can all can play a significant part in making it so. What follows are a few ways how.

Give credit where credit is due. As I discussed in Chapter 2, women want and deserve credit for the work of birth. As many before me have noted, doctors and midwives don't deliver babies—women do. We attend their deliveries, we assist them, but we don't deliver babies unless they are our own. This is true whatever the delivery mode, whether forceps or a cesarean is needed. The tools we use to help babies out of women's bodies are forms of assistance.

What does this mean? First, we should acknowledge our role as assistants when we talk to one another. We should talk not about "doing deliveries" but about "attending deliveries" or "attending women in birth." We should also acknowledge our role as assistants when we speak to our patients. When women thank us for what we do, we should first emphasize their own central role in the process and only then tell them they are welcome (or that we are honored), but that they are the deliverer, and we only catch or tug.

I understand that attending deliveries is hard work—no doubt we have weathered clogs and perhaps some strained relationships to show for it. But acknowledging the woman as the deliverer puts her back in the center of the drama that is birth, where she belongs. We cannot simply blame the mommy wars on the guilt that pervades women's post-birth assessments; providers have a role. You may find it confusing or sad that a woman could feel ashamed that she somehow "failed" even though she gave birth to a healthy baby. Giving credit where credit is due acknowledges the work that a woman has done in gestating and delivering a child—vaginally or by cesarean—and can help her recognize and feel proud of her role in birth.

Connect with your patient. What I heard from women time and again was that feeling emotionally connected to health care providers was an important part of a good birth. For most women, the detached but competent physician doesn't pass muster and can feel like a stranger, out of place. Many told us, rather, that what made their birth good was how intimate it felt, partly because of how deeply connected they felt to their midwife or doctor. No doubt the maternity care system can make it hard to get to know patients, but it's worth a try. Indeed, we heard scores of stories about how the requisite intimacy can be forged even in the space of a delivery.

Get moms and babies together quickly, but don't force first moments. For the most part, the women of the Good Birth Project appreciated—relished—the chance to see their babies soon after birth. When circumstances prevented their reconnecting quickly, the time that passed was remembered with regret, a dark hole in their childbirth experience. But different women had different needs once they got their first glimpse, their first sniff of their newborn's head. Some couldn't look away; others, though, really wanted a moment or two to get cleaned up, get settled, feel composed and calm enough to hold their child. No doubt maternity care practices have moved in the right direction in getting moms and babies together quickly. But it is nevertheless important to follow a woman's lead—get a sense from her about what she needs in the moment, whether it's uninterrupted contact or a few moments to regroup before taking on the mantle of "mommy."

Second, remember that for the most part, birth from women's perspectives is not just an arrival. As poets and writers and the women of the Good Birth Project have all noted, birth is an occasion for separation as well as attachment. Though we greet our newborns with delight, we also feel them leave, and feel with some trepidation the space between ourselves and our children. As we consider the etiology of and approaches to ongoing challenges, like the blues and depression too many women encounter after birth, it is worth considering that what happens in birth is not just an arrival, but the rending and re-forming of one of life's most intimate connections.

Words matter, so speak with care. As I listened to women, I was struck by the permanence of words uttered in delivery rooms. The majority of women we interviewed quoted someone—a doctor, midwife, nurse—noting what they said, how it made them feel, how the words continue to mark their birth for better or worse. What you say matters, endures, in ways you might never imagine. The words that cross your lips may be recounted time and again—across decades of a woman's life. The most memorable utterances tended not to be grand statements, but what you might think of as small things—words to which you might not give a second thought.

No doubt some of what will endure are well-intentioned but insensitive comments. Mother of six Jen recalled for us, after her second birth, her doctor saying, "That sure would have been easier if you'd had an epidural." When we asked her to tell us how the comment made her feel, she said, "It made me feel like throwing something at him . . . I felt confident, you know. I don't need an epidural—leave me alone . . . But then for the doctor to cut in with something, break my peace like that." You may still think (even correctly) that a birth would have been easier with an epidural. But don't say it while your patient is reveling in her achievement.

Several women talked about how important words of affirmation were to them. Mother of three Audra told us how she pressed across the threshold of transition, how she relied on the assurances of her midwife, who told her, "You're doing beautifully." Audra reflected that it was "all I needed to hear, the simplest thing. I just needed to hear that." Mother of two Cara felt the same way about her midwife telling her, "You can do it." She told us the words mattered, immensely. "I think all I needed was somebody to say, 'You can do it.' Like somebody in the medical establishment."

Of course, there is no script and the same words will strike different women differently. But respect, which I described in Chapter 5, can be a useful guidepost. In writing that chapter, I found I had to acknowledge time and again that women cannot control what other people do or say, that they may have to brace for disrespectful behavior. But *we* can control what we say, and our words do matter. Considering birth, the woman, and the baby as respectworthy, even sacred, will take us a long way in discerning when and how to speak.

Don't treat birth as a mere medical event. Some births are and should be medical events, to be sure. But all births are events that extend beyond the biological or medical—that have social, even existential meaning for women and families. And sociologists have shown how our culture regards pregnancy and birth as sacred events. For that reason, medical competence, while absolutely necessary, is not sufficient to your role in birth. Patients say that in birth they need more.

What this means is that getting a baby out safely is not the whole of your job. Women need those who attend them in birth to treat the event as something special, something sacred even. This doesn't mean you need to call in the chaplain. It simply means that you need to acknowledge that birth is an event that many of us set off from the mundane, the everyday. If you think of birth this way, it might help you anticipate the words and actions that are most likely to foster a good birth for your patient. We all appreciate what the offense would be of checking the score of a game or talking about some other patient while someone is exiting the world. Childbearing women tell us that the same sort of due regard is required when someone is entering the world as well.

There are countless ways that due regard can be realized. For one, don't rush your patient. Laboring women hate to be put on someone else's clock. It came as a surprise to me that several women said predictions about birth were off-putting. I'd often thought of them as a helpful means to give women a sense in real time of what they might expect in the hours ahead. But many women told us they want to labor on their own clock, be trusted about their own sense of progress—and that our projections can undermine their feelings of safety and confidence. Second, don't treat certain sorts of births as more respect-worthy than others. I'll get more specific about this below.

Cesarean birth should not require an apology. I'm not saying you shouldn't acknowledge a woman's disappointment—if she is disappointed—in having a surgical birth. But I'd offer, unless you've made a medical error, apologies have no place on a gurney en route to surgery, across a blue drape, in a postpartum room, or elsewhere. A cesarean is a birth. It is not a failure. Perhaps it feels like a failure on your part—a failed effort to avoid surgical birth, to keep the cesarean rate down where you or our profession thinks the cesarean rate should be. But a cesarean delivery marks the birth of a child, the birth of someone's child, and for that reason it is something not to apologize for but to celebrate.

Even when we don't use the words "I'm sorry," there are things we do in hospitals that communicate the notion of failure. Too many obstetricians and attendants go into "surgery mode" and stop thinking about the woman once she is belly-up on the table. I take as evidence of this signs in operating rooms on Labor and Delivery that remind personnel that "the patient is awake." If our behaviors in the operating rooms are so ingrained, the signs should also remind us that "The patient is giving birth. Tell her she's fantastic and her baby is beautiful. Congratulate her." Further, policies that keep women who have given birth vaginally in spacious LDRPs but wheel women post-cesarean to smaller rooms can communicate failure even when none is implied. Efforts in some hospitals to get women back into the LDRP she started in have been an important step toward keeping the spirit of celebration alive in surgical birth.

There is more we can do, like making the experience of cesarean better for women and their partners in the operating room. For instance, a group of doctors from the UK and Australia have pioneered a technique they (controversially—and unfortunately) call "natural cesarean." It entails early skin-to-skin contact, a slower more "physiological" delivery, and most important to my way of thinking, "engaging the parents as active participants in the birth of their child." Doctors led by anesthesiologist William Camann at Brigham and Women's Hospital in Boston have picked up on this and offer women clear surgical drapes so they can actually see their baby emerge through their abdominal incision. Notably, the Boston group uses instead the term "family-centered cesarean," which helpfully highlights the experience and values of the woman and her partner rather than "naturalness" of the process as a central goal. The often stark walls of the operating room need not preclude joy—it's time we figure out how best to make cesareans not just safe, but *good*.

There are also things done outside hospitals that link cesareans to failure. Cesareans no doubt get a bad rap in the media, are portrayed as evidence of obstetrical overreach, and are viewed primarily as something to be avoided rather than something that helps women deliver their children safely. What often fails to be acknowledged is that the majority of cesareans are still indicated and—yes—therapeutic. Many, in fact, are lifesaving.

This is not to say that you should dismiss a woman's feelings of loss from a cesarean. Quite the contrary. In fact, there is considerable harm in dismissing the loss some women feel in delivering their child through a surgical incision. Some women told us they needed to grieve their cesarean and wanted people to respect their need to do so, even though they had a healthy baby in arms. There is a big difference between acknowledging a loss (cesarean can feel like one) and conceptualizing an event as a "failure."

One last observation: In addition to having doctors and midwives who knew how to keep the spirit of celebration, and sometimes sanctity, alive, there was something else that helped women push back against the notion of failure when things like unplanned cesarean or hospital transfer occurred. It was feeling assured that what happened was necessary. They wanted to feel like every stone was left unturned, that they were given every chance of having the sort of delivery they wanted. An eleven-pound baby could serve as evidence, as could some tangible proof of pathology like a knot in the cord or an occult abruption. If a cesarean is required—by a knot or dystocia or any number of issues that would prevent a safe birth—there is no reason for apology. Assure your patient—if you can—that your intervention was needed. Then tell her congratulations, for becoming a mother, for delivering her child beautifully.

Remember that birth always occurs in the context of someone's life. Women bring their lives to birth, their attachments and hopes. Decisions about and responses to birthing often reach beyond risk numbers, through which we doctors often sift, beyond clinical findings and markers of reassurance or concern. Some of your patients will let you in on these things and give you a sense of what moves them and why; others will not. It's worth lending an ear, I daresay even lengthening obstetrical appointments, to make room for life stories in the context of care.

Midwife Donna recalled for us births—we've all seen them—where "you knew something was holding things up." Not a small pelvis or a big baby—but something else, something tugging on a woman's heart or life. Such was the case for her patient Janine who was transferred—fully dilated—from birthing center to hospital, at Janine's own urgent request. She pushed her child out within minutes of being tucked into a hospital bed. Later, she reminded Donna that she'd originally been carrying twins and one had died early on, and she just "didn't feel ready to meet this new baby because she hadn't really felt like she'd said good-bye to the one that wasn't being born."

And of course births can be shaped profoundly by events outside the birthing room that seem at first glance if important, unrelated. For instance, mother of two Rose lost her father in the interim between the births of her two children. The best part about her second birth was having a nurse with whom she could "talk openly about how sad it was that my dad wasn't there." Otherwise, she told us, the process, the birth—even with the blessing of a healthy baby, "would have been really sad." Simone, described in Chapter 4, noted she lost her grandmother at the same time she delivered her first child— a preamble, perhaps, to the postpartum darkness she endured. This is all to say that births are enmeshed with lives—and we all need to look beyond risk numbers and clinical indicators to understand women's choices and experiences, to help them get to the good in birth.

Do not presume that your ideal is the ideal. In this conception of a good birth, based on diverse women's views, it is clear that there are many ways to find value and meaning in birth. Indeed, time and again I discovered many pathways to the same end. Presence could be achieved by the concentration that unanesthetized birth requires, or by an epidural that keeps "distracting" pain at bay. Feelings of security could be found in homes and hospitals. I could go on. What I want to emphasize, though, is that we distilled a notion of a good birth across many kinds of births and circumstances. You may have experienced or attended a birth that struck you as good— even ideal. But honoring birth and honoring women requires acknowledging that there is not a single ideal—that there is a breadth of good births. We should take seriously women's values and experiences and shape maternity care and dialogue, not to press a single ideal, but to accommodate good births in all their variation.

In deciding how to measure the quality of maternity care, women's views should take center stage. As the health care system is changing, so will our approach to maternity care. Women's voices and preferences need a bigger role.

As the women of the Good Birth Project attest, physical health, although deeply valued, is a crude and insensitive marker of the degree to which a birth was good. Similarly, the presence or absence of technological intervention doesn't capture what women say matters most. As such, it would be misleading to limit measures of quality to discrete health outcomes; likewise, it would be misleading to evaluate quality according to how much technology was used. We shouldn't count epidurals as a negative "complication" of birth, when the majority of women who used epidurals valued them and could articulate myriad ways in which they contributed to a good birth experience. Measures of quality must reflect the things that matter most to patients, the women we serve.

We need to seriously reconsider our approach to birth, the ways we think and talk about it, the frames through which we measure success. Birth is an extraordinary event in the lives of women, indeed in all our lives.

A Good Birth lays the groundwork for a robust notion of appropriate and worthy ends in birth, ends to which we all can and should aspire. Childbearing women will show us the way.

Acknowledgments

Whatever made me think that the right time to write my first book was in the first year of my fourth child's life I will never know. But it turned out to be, and I am grateful for everyone who, without questioning the wisdom of the undertaking, helped make it happen.

I am extremely grateful to Bill Shinker and Lauren Marino for taking on *A Good Birth*, for believing in it, and me. At Avery, it has been my privilege to work with Marisa Vigilante and her stellar team. Marisa's careful, elegant editing, her patience and gentle treatment of a sensitive (and passionate) author, and her enduring enthusiasm for the project have made the process a pleasure.

On Mother's Day 2011, I received an e-mail from Gail Ross, who became my agent, with the subject line "I love this project" and a note that she'd intentionally waited until the notable holiday, until after she'd talked to her daughters, to read my book proposal. I was (and am) smitten, and am deeply grateful to Gail for all she has done. She threw herself behind me and the book, unflinchingly pressed us forward as I rounded the last trimester of pregnancy, then coaxed me out of the rocking chair when Will was weeks old to join her on a whirlwind tour of New York publishing houses, ultimately finding me a home at Avery and Penguin. I am also grateful to Howard Yoon, Gail's partner at the Ross Yoon agency, for not letting up on the hard questions, and to Anna Sproul for her careful attention to my project.

It has been said (and I believe it to be true, in many ways) that writing and birthing are similar undertakings. If this is the case, Jenna Free is the best midwife the editing world has to offer. Her help as I wrote was indispensable—sometimes gentle, encouraging, and empathic, but tough as nails too when the project and process demanded it, especially when I needed to work through those last tough contractions (chapters). She dove deep with me and encouraged me to go deeper, unflinchingly identified errors in prose and logic, and helped me see the coherent whole. Thank you, Jenna, from the bottom of my heart.

I am grateful to Sarah Flynn for helping me out of the gate to understand what it would take to write a serious book about birth for the women and men I aimed to reach, for connecting me with Gail, and for being a source of wisdom through the process. I'm also grateful to my Chapel Hill writing group—Paula Michaels, Sarah Shields, Gigi Dillon, and Emily Burrill—who with the right combination of empathy and toughness helped me get my book proposal in shape to send out, and muster the courage to do it.

I cannot imagine having written *A Good Birth* absent the friendship and generosity—intellectual and otherwise—of Maggie Little, confidant, critic (in the best, most crucial sense of the word), and simply one of my favorite women alive. Much of my current thinking on reproduction came out of years of conversations with Maggie and an extraordinary group of women we brought together in 2004: Betsy Armstrong, Rebecca Kukla, Miriam Kuppermann, Lisa Mitchell, and Lisa Harris. I owe each and all a depth of gratitude, and am particularly grateful to Lisa Harris and Maggie for their careful reading and honest commentary on drafts of the manuscript, for affirming my vision and revealing my blind spots, for sharing so much of their time and their brilliant selves.

Ruth Faden—mentor, colleague, dear friend—has been a major inspiration throughout the project, from the first moment I mentioned it to her ("You must do this, Annie," she said; I still have my notes from that call—"I must do this," I wrote). Ruth's brilliance and elegance and way of seeing the world have helped me see who I want to be and what I want to contribute. I could almost hear her voice as I wrote the book. Thank you, dear Ruth, for believing.

I could not have conducted the Good Birth Project without the generous support of the Greenwall Foundation. I am particularly indebted to Bill Stubing, who always seemed to understand the resonance between birth and death and always seemed to know I'd get this book written. My experiences as a Fellow and Scholar gave me the courage to ask "big" questions, and a diverse network of amazingly smart and thoughtful colleagues willing to consider and critique my efforts to answer them. I am grateful to Alisa Carse at Georgetown, who originally helped me home in on the lacuna that drove my inquiry. My deep gratitude also extends to the advisory board of the Scholars program—Bernie Lo, Christine Cassel, Baruch Brody, and Jim Curran. Karla Holloway cheered me on, braced me for the journey, shared elation across the hurdles as only someone who has been through it—and loves language and books as I do—could. My conversations with Bo Burt attuned me to the deep questions upon which I was pressing; those conversations and feedback on the manuscript made me think harder, and work harder to get to heart of the matter, making it a much better book. I am also grateful to many of the diverse and brilliant Greenwall Fellows and Faculty Scholars, who never let up in their interest or anticipation.

For the substantial work of conducting and analyzing data for the Good Birth Project, I am grateful to my research team and the incredibly thoughtful and careful leadership of Emily Namey. Emily put her heart into the project, conducted exquisite interviews, helped me sift through mountains of gorgeous data, listened hard. Well more than an extraordinary research associate, you are a dear friend. Thanks also to others on our research team, particularly Natasha Mack and Brownsyne Tucker-Edmonds.

What also made the book possible was getting a dream job, with dream bosses and colleagues at the University of North Carolina at Chapel Hill School of Medicine. Gail Henderson and Eric Juengst have been unwaveringly supportive of the project, with the perfect combination of flexibility, expectation, and enthusiasm. I am grateful for wonderful conversations with my colleagues in the Department of Social Medicine and Center for Bioethics, particularly Rebecca Walker, Mara Buchbinder, Anna Brandon, and Deborah Porterfield, as well as the constant stimulation that comes from being surrounded by such an extraordinary and diverse group of thoughtful scholars.

The Trent Center for Bioethics, Humanities & History of Medicine at Duke was a wonderful space to conduct the Good Birth Project, and I am grateful to colleagues there for their support in the project's formative years. Working (and gabbing) with the deft and empathic Sally Howland in the Duke Miscarriage Clinic was immensely enlightening (and enjoyable) and has helped me understand birth's relationship to loss in a way I never could have before.

I was extremely fortunate to connect with a trio of visionaries in the world of midwifery: Kitty Ernst, Ruth Lubic, and Maureen Darcey. I am grateful to each for trusting a curious doctor, sharing their wisdom and time, and swinging open the doors of the spaces they'd created to help women find their way to a good birth. I learned so much from each of you. Thank you. I am also grateful to Phyllis Leppert for understanding what I was up to and thinking to connect me with Kitty and Ruth.

Several of my colleagues in obstetrics have also shaped in profound ways my thinking on birth, most particularly Andra James and Elizabeth Livingston—but also so many of the doctors and nurses with whom I trained and worked and who helped me see and aspire to the best sort of care for women with the full range of health needs.

At the heart of this book are the voices of more than a hundred women who participated in the Good Birth Project. I am grateful to each for speaking so generously and thoughtfully, for offering insight and stories that moved us to tears, that surprised us, that helped us see birth in new and important ways. Your words and wisdom have brought these pages to life. Thank you. I am also grateful to the maternity care providers we interviewed for their honesty and insight, for responding with whole hearts. You give me faith that the sort of progress we need to make is well within reach. I owe a special debt to the countless women (and men)—some friends, others relative strangers—who openly shared their thoughts and experiences about birth, at coffee shops and parties and in school pickup lines and park benches and doorways that welcomed sometimes intimate conversations. Your stories and wisdom also line these pages. Thank you.

In carving a space to do the work this book required in the chaos of my life, I relied and am grateful for the support and enthusiasm of several dear friends, notably Betsy and John Pringle, Susan Gravely and Bill Ross, Joanie Preyer, and Lisa Kang. Our Sunday walks, Lisa, gave me the courage and reassurance I needed to write on so many Monday mornings. I am also grateful for the forbearance of some of my oldest and dearest friends, for the unspoken assurance that you'd be there for me when I surfaced again, the forgiveness for missed celebrations and get-togethers: among them, Sally Barry, Melanie DeMonet, Amy Groff, Shirley TerMolen, and Astrid Womble.

Brenda Guittierez took such good and confident care of William while I wrote, especially during our first weeks (well, months) home from the hospital, that I was able to focus even in those early and intense days of new motherhood. I was never one to write with a baby stretched across my lap, and I could never have sunk into the book if I didn't know Will and his brothers were in the safest and most loving of hands nearby. I knew they were (and are) with you. *Gracias.*

Most of all, I thank my family: my mom, whose wisdom runs like threads through the book and my life, who is always there, believing and cheering on, sending love and providing support. I feel unimaginably lucky to be your daughter.

That I learned, on the same day, of both my first pregnancy and my father's imminently life-ending stroke could be understood as a cruel coincidence, though it never struck me that way. I do regret, and deeply, that he never got to meet my children, his grandchildren. But as a force in my life he endures, and this book attests in large part to what he taught me when he was alive and the meaning I've found in his early departure. There is no doubt in my mind that his reflections on our births catapulted me toward the work I do, toward the question at the heart of this book, emboldened by the confidence that came of being my father's daughter.

I am deeply grateful to both Diane and Tanna Drapkin, for so generously sharing the stories around their births, for opening my heart and mind further to the wisdom of midwifery from the standpoint of women, and for their enthusiasm and sisterhood through the process of researching and writing. I am also grateful to my brothers, Mike and Steve Drapkin, for bringing such extraordinary and wise women into our circle and for giving me the sisters I never imagined I'd have (and for being great brothers to boot). I am also grateful to Josie Becker for getting how important and challenging this has been for me, for the constant offering of good wishes (and good snacks). You are a beloved Auntie and kindred spirit.

I could not have written this book without the enduring support of my husband, Kim (in birth and afterward), his brilliant insights, his open heart, his unsounded patience, his inspiring tenacity, his unwavering belief that I could do it—and the inimitable twinkle in his eye that made me believe it too. You are the love of my life, and our fortune in finding each other never ceases to amaze me.

Finally, thanks to my darling boys, Grant, Paul, Charlie, and Will, for waiting patiently on the big white chair when I had to get that last sentence out, for asking me and wanting to know how the book was going, for wrapping your arms around me and each other, for the countless ways in which you are utterly riveting to your mom. And dear Gracie, who came into our lives just as I heaved the sigh of relief that comes with finishing the endeavor that is a book—your timing was exquisite, as are you. I love each of you— Grant, Paul, Charlie, Will, and Grace—with all my heart.

Appendix

Characteristics of Women Who Participated in the Good Birth Project						
Characteristic	"Wise Women" (Multiparas)* (n=62)		First-Time Moms (Primiparas)* (n=39)		Total (n=101)	
	n	%	n	%	n	%
Age in years—average						
At interview	31		29		30	
At first birth	26		29		28	
Race						
African-American	19	31%	10	26%	29	29%
Asian	3	5%	5	13%	8	8%
European-American	31	50%	18	46%	49	49%
Hispanic	6	10%	6	15%	12	12%
Mixed/Other	3	5%	0	0%	3	3%
Education						
Some high school	8	13%	2	5%	10	10%
High school degree	5	8%	4	10%	9	9%
Some college	8	13%	4	10%	12	12%
College degree	21	34%	10	26%	31	32%
Graduate degree	20	32%	17	44%	37	37%

Previously published in "The Meaning of 'Control' for Childbearing Women in the U.S." by Emily Namey and Anne Drapkin Lyerly, *Social Science and Medicine* 71 (2010): 769-76.

Characteristics of Women Who Participated in the Good Birth Project, continued						
Characteristic	*"Wise Women" (Multiparas)* (n=62)*		*First-Time Moms (Primiparas)* (n=39)*		*Total (n=101)*	
	n	*%*	*n*	*%*	*n*	*%*
Annual household income						
<$20K	10	16%	6	15%	16	16%
$20K–50K	12	19%	8	21%	20	20%
$50K–100K	18	29%	10	26%	28	28%
>$100K	19	31%	12	31%	31	31%
Married	46	74%	30	77%	76	75%
Total births	162		39		201	
Births per woman (average)	2.6		1			
Births per woman (range)	2–7		1			
At least one high-risk pregnancy	25	40%	6	15%	31	31%
At least one cesarean delivery	24	39%	13	33%	37	37%
Location of delivery†						
Hospital	52	84%	25	64%	77	76%
Birth center	14	23%	6	15%	20	20%
Home	10	16%	3	8%	13	13%
Mode of delivery†						
Vaginal	48	77%	22	56%	70	69%
VBAC	7	11%	0	0%	7	7%
Planned cesarean	10	16%	5	13%	15	15%
Unplanned cesarean	19	31%	8	21%	27	27%

NOTE: Rows within a category may not add up to 100 percent, as not all participants answered every question, and five first-time moms were lost to follow-up before their postpartum interview.

*The term multiparas is the medical word for women who have given birth more than once (our already "wise women"); the term primiparas is the medical term for women who are giving birth for the first time, or who have given birth to one child (our "first-time moms").

†Numbers and percentages included in these rows reflect the number of *women* in our sample who experienced at least one birth in this setting or via this mode of delivery; women with multiple birth experiences are potentially counted in more than one category.

Notes on Sources

Introduction: In Search of a Good Birth

Page 1   "Only when the conscious experience of mothers": Virginia Held, "Birth and Death," *Ethics* 99, 2 (1989): 388.

Page 1   "It is important to remember": Adrienne Rich, *Of Woman Born: Motherhood as Experience and Institution* (New York: W. W. Norton, 1995), 130.

Page 3   These two views of birth: Barbara Katz Rothman, *In Labor: Women and Power in the Birthplace* (New York: W. W. Norton, 1991); see also Robbie Davis-Floyd, *Birth as an American Rite of Passage*, 2nd ed. (Berkeley: University of California Press, 2004); and Judith Rooks, *Midwifery and Childbirth in America* (Philadelphia: Temple University Press, 1997).

Page 5   Take for instance the tale of Elizabeth Rourke: Atul Gawande, "The Score: How Childbirth Went Industrial," *The New Yorker*, October 9, 2006.

Page 7   consider the "Optimality Index": "Measuring Outcomes of Midwifery Care: The Optimality Index—U.S.," http://www.midwife.org/Optimality-Index-US.

Page 8   as historians note was common at the time: Jacqueline H. Wolf, *Deliver Me from Pain: Anesthesia and Birth in America* (Baltimore: The Johns Hopkins University Press, 2012).

Page 8   the unreflective use of external fetal monitoring: Z. Alfirevic, D. Devane, and G. M. Gyte, "Continuous Cardiotocography (CTG) as a Form of Electronic Fetal Monitoring (EFM) for Fetal Assessment During Labor," *Cochrane Database of Systematic Reviews* 19, 3 (2006); see also Alastair MacLennan, Karin B. Nelson, and Gary Hankins, "Who Will Deliver Our Grandchildren?" *Journal of the American Medical Association* 294 (2005): 1688–90.

Page 10   "it was as if the phenomena did not actually exist": Ira Byock, *Dying Well* (New York: Riverhead Books, 1998), 31.

Page 11   "When the human dimension of dying is nurtured": Ibid., 57.

Page 11   the goal is not an idealized or scripted death: See, e.g., Henry Perkins, "Controlling Death: The False Promise of Advance Directives," *Annals of Internal Medicine* 147 (2007): 51–57.

Page 13   Inspired by psychologist Carol Gilligan's work on moral development: Carol Gilligan, *In a Different Voice: Psychological Theory and Women's Development* (Cambridge, Mass.: Harvard University Press, 1982).

Page 13   Things we doctors and midwives see as central points of contention: See, e.g., Childbirth Connection: *Listening to Mothers* Surveys and Reports, available at http://www .childbirthconnection.org/article.asp?ClickedLink=334&ck=10068&area=27

Page 14   Additional details of how we designed and carried out the study: Emily Namey and Anne Drapkin Lyerly, "The Meaning of 'Control' for Childbearing Women in the U.S.," *Social Science and Medicine* 71 (2010): 769–76.

Page 15   new accounts of well-being: Madison Powers and Ruth Faden, *Social Justice: The Moral Foundations of Public Health* (New York: Oxford University Press, 2006).

Page 17   In 1985, esteemed professor of public health Allan Rosenfield: Allan Rosenfield and Deborah Maine, "Maternal Mortality—A Neglected Tragedy: Where Is the M in MCH?" *The Lancet* 2, 8446 (1985): 83–85.

Page 17   Faden called attention to the fact: Ruth Faden, Nancy Kass, and Deven McGraw, "Women as Vessels and Vectors: Lessons from the HIV Epidemic," in Susan Wolf, ed., *Feminism and Bioethics: Beyond Reproduction*, 252–81 (New York: Oxford University Press, 1996).

Page 17   In 2008, the National Institutes of Health rolled out a major study: Anne Drapkin Lyerly, Margaret Olivia Little, and Ruth Faden, "The National Children's Study: A Golden Opportunity to Advance the Health of Pregnant Women," *American Journal of Public Health* 99, 10 (2009): 1742–45.

Page 18   other researchers and scholars have made progress in this regard: Judith Walzer Leavitt, *Make Room for Daddy: The Journey from Waiting Room to Birthing Room* (Chapel Hill: University of North Carolina Press, 2009); see also Martha Montello, "Being There," *Current Problems in Pediatric and Adolescent Health Care* 41 (2011): 109–10.

Page 18   "I think of my children's births—carry them around with me—every day of my life": Joyce Maynard, *Domestic Affairs: Enduring the Pleasures of Motherhood and Family Life* (New York: Crown, 1987).

Page 19   Penny Simkin actually studied women's memories: Penny Simkin, "Just Another Day in a Woman's Life? Women's Long-Term Perceptions of Their First Birth Experience," Part 1, *Birth* 18, 4 (1991): 203–10; and Penny Simkin, "Just Another Day in a Woman's Life? Nature and Consistency of Women's Long-Term Memories of Their First Birth Experience," *Birth* 19, 2 (1992): 64–81.

Page 20   "both a paradigm and parable": Louise Erdrich, *The Blue Jay's Dance: A Memoir of Early Motherhood* (New York: HarperCollins, 1995), 44.

Page 21   their impact on the health care system is significant: C. DeFrances, C. Lucas, V. Buie, and A. Golosinskiy, Division of Health Care Statistics, "2006 National Hospi-

tal Discharge Survey," *National Health Statistics Reports* (2008), http://www.cdc
.gov/nchs/data/nhsr/nhsr005.pdf; see also "HCUPnet, Healthcare Cost and Utili-
zation Project," Agency for Healthcare Research and Quality, Rockville, MD (2008),
www.hcupnet.ahrq.gov.

One: Control

Page 25   "Perhaps my greatest stroke of luck": Susan Maushart, *The Mask of Motherhood: How
Becoming a Mother Changes Our Lives and Why We Never Talk About It* (New York:
Penguin Books, 1999), 96.

Page 25   "There are certain frustrations in approaching such an event": Erdrich, 43.

Page 26   found control and childbirth satisfaction to be strongly related: Ellen Hodnett, "Pain
and Women's Satisfaction with the Experience of Childbirth: A Systematic Review,"
American Journal of Obstetrics & Gynecology 186, 5, supplement (2002): S160–72.

Page 38   the "masculine weapon" in the public struggle: Rich, 146.

Page 38   "superiority and control of Male over Female, Technology over Nature": Davis-
Floyd, 130.

Page 40   birth is a considerably safer endeavor . . . than it was a hundred years ago: Judith
Walzer Leavitt, *Brought to Bed: Childbearing in America, 1750–1950* (New York: Oxford University Press, 1986).

Page 40   the actual numbers may not correlate so neatly: Ibid., 28.

Page 41   medicine "attracts people with high personal anxieties about dying": Sherwin Nuland, *How We Die: Reflections on Life's Final Chapter* (New York: Vintage, 1993), 258.

Page 43   "ruthlessly yanking Linus's blanket away from him": Michael Green quoted by Denise Grady, in "Oxygen Monitor Fails to Help Doctors Detect Birth Defects," *The
New York Times*, November 23, 2006.

Page 43   the best studies show that just listening: Alfirevic et al.

Page 43   Much has been made . . . of the human tendency toward "magical thinking": See,
e.g., Matthew Hutson, *The 7 Laws of Magical Thinking: How Irrational Beliefs Keep Us
Happy, Healthy, and Sane* (New York: Hudson Street Press, 2012).

Page 46   the women of the Good Birth Project really wanted something specific . . . when
they said they wanted "control": Namey and Lyerly.

Two: Agency

Page 49   "I had to figure out how to push hard enough": Faulkner Fox, *Dispatches from a
Not-So-Perfect Life* (New York: Broadway, 2004), 91.

Page 49   "But who gives it? And to whom is it given?": Margaret Atwood, "Giving Birth," in
Dancing Girls and Other Stories (Toronto: McClelland and Stewart, 1977).

Page 53   [epidurals] have no effect on the risk of cesarean section or the health of newborns:
M. Anim-Somuah, R. M. Smith, and L. Jones, "Epidural Versus Non-Epidural or
No Analgesia in Labour," *Cochrane Database of Systematic Reviews* 7, 12 (2011).

Page 54   they work better than the alternatives: L. Jones et al., "Pain Management for Women
in Labour: An Overview of Systematic Reviews," *Cochrane Database of Systematic
Reviews* 14, 3 (2012).

Page 59   "When the *doctor* is delivering the baby": Rothman, 174.

Page 59   "When I boast to friends that I delivered our baby": William Sears and Martha Sears, *The Baby Book: Everything You Need to Know About Your Baby from Birth to Age Two* (New York: Little, Brown, 1993), 41–42.

Page 63   A paper I love: Hilde Lindemann Nelson, "The Architect and the Bee: Some Reflections on Postmortem Pregnancy," *Bioethics* 8, 3 (1994): 247–67.

Page 67   bearing witness "exceeds seeing": Sue Tait, "Bearing Witness: Journalism and Moral Responsibility," *Media, Culture and Society* 33, 8 (2011): 1220–35.

Page 71   the *American Journal of Obstetrics & Gynecology* published a major systematic review: Hodnett, S160.

Three: Personal Security

Page 75   "Ambiguous things can seem very threatening": Mary Douglas, *Purity and Danger* (London: Routledge Classics, 2002), xi.

Page 75   "During idylls of safety": Diane Ackerman, "The Brain on Love," *The New York Times*, March 24, 2012.

Page 76   One study showed that even if everyone with a baby north of nine pounds had a cesarean: D. H. Delpapa and E. Mueller-Heubach, "Pregnancy Outcome Following Ultrasound Diagnosis of Macrosomia," *Obstetrics and Gynecology* 78 (1991): 340–43.

Page 76   you'd still likely have to do thousands of otherwise unnecessary cesareans: D. J. Rouse et al., "The Effectiveness and Costs of Elective Cesarean Delivery for Fetal Macrosomia Diagnosed by Ultrasound," *Journal of the American Medical Association* 276 (1996): 1480–86; the article estimates that 2,345 extra cesareans would have to be done to prevent one permanent injury.

Page 77   a policy of preemptive cesareans isn't appropriate: Robert J. Sokol and Sean C. Blackwell for the ACOG Committee on Practice Bulletins, Practice Bulletin #40: *Shoulder Dystocia* (2010), http://www.acog.org/Resources_And_Publications /Practice_Bulletins/Committee_on_Practice_Bulletins_Obstetrics/Shoulder _Dystocia.

Page 77   according to a couple of well-done studies: Suneet P. Chauhan et al., "Rapid Estimation of Birth Weights: Ask the Mother," *The New England Journal of Medicine* 326 (1992): 1504; see also S. P. Chauhan et al., "Intrapartum Clinical, Sonographic and Parous Patients' Estimates of Newborn Birth Weight," *Obstetrics and Gynecology* 79, 6 (1992): 956–58.

Page 79   "human interests everyone has": Powers and Faden, 18.

Page 81   There is some consensus: NIH Consensus Development Conference on "Vaginal Birth After Cesarean: New Insights," March 8–10, 2010. Final Panel Statement available at http://consensus.nih.gov/2010/vbacstatement.htm. See also Anne Drapkin Lyerly and Margaret Olivia Little, "Toward an Ethical Approach to Vaginal Birth After Cesarean," *Seminars in Perinatology* 34 (2010): 337–44.

Page 87   consumer advocates press hospitals to be more transparent: See, e.g., Cesarean -rates.com.

Page 87   The Institute of Medicine estimated: Linda T. Kohn, Janet M. Corrigan, and Molla S. Donald, eds., Committee on Quality Health Care in America, *To Err Is Human: Building a Safer Health System* (Washington, D.C.: National Academies Press, 1999).

Page 89   "Once you've been on the losing side of great odds": Elizabeth McCracken, *An Exact Replica of a Figment of My Imagination* (New York: Little, Brown, 2008), 115.

Page 99   It is a term evoked by "father of modern medicine" and Johns Hopkins professor: William Osler, "Aequanimitas," valedictory address, University of Pennsylvania, May 1, 1889, available at http://www.medicalarchives.jhmi.edu/osler/aequessay.htm.

Page 101   in her recent book *Pushed*: Jennifer Block, *Pushed: The Painful Truth About Childbirth and Modern Maternity Care* (Cambridge, Mass.: Da Capo Lifelong, 2007).

Page 107   "Though we seek to create order": Douglas, 117.

Page 108   "Dangers . . . are manifold and omnipresent": Ibid., xix.

Four: Connectedness

Page 111   "Here, under my heart": Erica Jong, "The Birth of the Water Baby" (excerpt), available at http://www.ericajong.com/poems/birthofwaterbaby.htm.

Page 119   Judith Rooks has for years championed making nitrous oxide available: Judith Rooks, "Use of Nitrous Oxide in Midwifery Practice—Complementary, Synergistic, and Needed in the United States," *Journal of Midwifery & Women's Health* 52 (2007): 186–89.

Page 120   It's come to hold a nearly magical aura . . . following an article: M. H. Klaus et al., "Maternal Attachment: Importance of the First Post-Partum Days," *The New England Journal of Medicine* 286, 9 (1972): 460–63.

Page 121   "Eight months with my son": Samantha Shapiro, "Mommy Wars, the Prequel: Ina May Gaskin and the Battle for At-Home Births," *The New York Times*, May 23, 2012.

Page 125   "To be pregnant is to be *inhabited*": Margaret Olivia Little, "Abortion, Intimacy, and the Duty to Gestate," *Ethical Theory and Moral Practice* 2 (1999): 301.

Page 126   a "harrowing experience" for babies: Sears, 41.

Page 141   Doctors, she argues, need two things: Jodi Halpern, "'Empathic Civilization': Why Empathy Is Essential for Doctors and in Conflict Resolution," *The Huffington Post*, February 23, 2010; see also Jodi Halpern, *From Detached Concern to Empathy* (New York: Oxford University Press, 2011).

Five: Respect

Page 155   "At last, with the birth of each daughter": Erdrich, 50.

Page 157   headline-grabbing $42 million gift: Dirk Johnson, "A $42 Million Gift Aims at Improving Bedside Manner," *The New York Times*, September 22, 2011.

Page 158   As many have noted to be true about the other bookend of life: See, e.g., Byock, 57.

Page 159   our culture and many others mark pregnancy and birth: Jane Balin, "The Sacred Dimensions of Pregnancy and Birth," *Qualitative Sociology* 11 (1988): 275–301.

Page 161   "drama of unprecedented power": Maushart, 72.

Page 165   Nearly seventy-five years ago: Michel Leiris, "The Sacred in Everyday Life," lecture to the Collège de Sociologie (1938), available at http://www.scribd.com/doc/59874791/Michael-Leiris-The-Sacred-in-Everyday-Life.

Page 166   NPR did a story on them: Andrea Hsu, "Born in the USA? This Blanket Might Look Familiar," June 22, 2011, available at http://www.npr.org/2011/07/22/138575125/born-in-the-usa-this-blanket-might-look-familiar.

Page 168   "prolonged effort will produce a kind of dazzled blindness": Robert A. Burt, *Death Is That Man Taking Names* (Berkeley: University of California Press, 2002), 4.

Page 181   "consider 'Is this the best forkful of food I can give my baby?'": Arlene Eisenberg, Heidi Murkoff, and Sandee Hathaway, *What to Expect When You're Expecting* (New York: Workman, 1996), 81; the phrase, though not the sentiment, is notably absent from more recent editions.

Page 185   "Your body is not a lemon!": Ina May Gaskin, *Ina May's Guide to Childbirth* (New York: Bantam, 2003).

Six: Knowledge

Page 191   "The majority of women, literate or illiterate": Rich, 157.

Page 191   "I have always been extremely fond of the definition of Death": Sylvia Plath, excerpt from "The Unabridged Journals of Sylvia Plath (1957–62)," in Moyra Davey, ed., *Mother Reader: Essential Literature on Motherhood*, 20 (New York: Seven Stories Press, 2011).

Page 194   more information is not always better: See, e.g., Sheena Iyengar, *The Art of Choosing* (New York: Twelve, 2010); and Alina Tugend, "Too Many Choices: A Problem That Can Paralyze, *The New York Times*, February 26, 2010.

Page 195   Most medications used during pregnancy have not been tested: Ruth Faden, Anne Drapkin Lyerly, and Maggie Little, "A Custom Drug," *The New York Times*, May 9, 2009; see also Francoise Baylis, "Pregnant Women Deserve Better," *Nature* 465 (2010): 689–90; Anne Drapkin Lyerly, Margaret Olivia Little, and Ruth Faden, "Pregnancy and Clinical Research," *Hastings Center Report* 38, 6 (2008); and Bonnie Rochman, "The Risks (and Rewards) of Pills and Pregnancy," *Time*, June 8, 2009.

Page 199   "women didn't really need to know about their bodies": Christine Cupaiuolo, in "Landmark Book on Women's Health Turns 40," NPR, October 13, 2011, available at http://www.npr.org/2011/10/13/141320033/landmark-book-on-womens-sexuality-turns-40. See the current edition, Boston Women's Health Book Collective, *Our Bodies, Ourselves* (New York: Touchstone, 2011).

Page 202   "battle-scarred, bewildered, and betrayed": Maushart, 64.

Seven: Looking Forward, Looking Back: Birth as Transformation

Page 221   "Whether figured as a death or heroic rebirth": Tess Cosslet, *Women Writing Childbirth: Modern Discourses of Motherhood* (New York: Manchester University Press, 1994), 154.

Page 221   "I have been asked if I had the choice again": Susan Griffin, "Feminism and Motherhood" (1974), in Davey, 34.

Page 224 ascribe Nancy's elation and acceptance followed by disappointment to the "halo effect": Simkin (1992), 70.

Page 227 Power . . . is usually thought of as the stuff of "female CEOs . . . and Hollywood mogulettes": Margaret Talbot, "In the Balance: Women and Power in 2001," *The New York Times Magazine*, September 9, 2001.

Epilogue: Common Ground: Notes to Maternity Care Providers

Page 240 In a letter to *The New York Times*: Katharine Wenstrom, "Mommy Wars: The Prequel" (letter), June 8, 2012.

Page 240 most obstetrical studies fail to consider a cesarean incision as injurious: Claire Wendland, "The Vanishing Mother: Cesarean Section and 'Evidence-Based Obstetrics,'" *Medical Anthropology Quarterly* 21, 2 (2007): 218–33.

Page 244 a group of doctors from the UK and Australia: J. Smith, F. Plaat and N. M. Fisk, "The Natural Cesarean: A Woman-Centred Technique," *British Journal of Obstetrics and Gynecology* 115, 8 (2008): 1037–42; see also William Camann and Robert Barbieri, "Mother-, Baby-, and Family-Centered Cesarean Delivery: It Is Possible," *OBG Management* 25, 3 (2013): 10, 12, 15.

Glossary

abruption: A complication of pregnancy in which the placenta separates prematurely from its point of attachment to the wall of the uterus. The condition usually results in bleeding and can be life-threatening for women and babies.

amniotic fluid: The fluid surrounding a fetus during pregnancy, contained by a thick membrane (the *amniotic sac*) often called the "bag of waters."

autonomy: The ability of each person to govern herself or her life, literally "self-rule." Respect for autonomy is a basic tenet of medical ethics.

birth center: Can refer to any facility dedicated to providing care for women giving birth. In this book, the term refers to freestanding "homelike" facilities that provide low-intervention maternity care by midwives. See www.birthcenters.org.

cervix: The opening to the uterus at the top of the vagina. Over the course of labor, the cervix dilates from zero to ten centimeters to allow for passage of the baby.

cesarean: Birth achieved through an incision in a woman's abdomen and uterus; also called a *cesarean section* or *C-section.*

doula (doo-lah)*:* A nonmedical person who assists a childbearing woman and her family by providing information, physical assistance, practical help, or emotional support before, during, or after delivery.

dystocia: A difficult or prolonged labor; often used to refer to *shoulder dystocia*, in which the anterior shoulder of the baby gets stuck behind a woman's pubic bone (after the baby's head has delivered), which is considered an obstetrical emergency. Doctors, midwives, and nurses are usually trained to perform a series of maneuvers to release the shoulder and effect safe delivery.

epidural: A form of anesthesia in which pain medicine is delivered by a thin tube to the space just outside the spinal canal, usually resulting in numbing from the woman's midsection down.

fetus: The technical term used for a human before birth, starting at eight weeks gestation. Some practitioners and patients will use and prefer the term "baby" in conversation.

forceps: The curved metal instruments resembling tongs that are sometimes placed around a baby's head, once it is low in the birth canal, to facilitate vaginal delivery. Forceps are occasionally used during cesarean.

Labor and Delivery: The name of the ward in most hospitals for women giving birth, sometimes called *L-and-D*.

maternal-fetal specialist: A physician who typically has three years of advanced training beyond general obstetrics and cares for women with medically complicated pregnancies; sometimes called a *perinatologist*.

meconium: Green or brown material staining the amniotic fluid. Meconium comes from a fetus defecating in the uterus and occurs in 8-20 percent of pregnancies. It is often considered a sign of stress but also occurs in uncomplicated labor. Meconium can get in the baby's lungs and cause breathing problems.

midwife: A practitioner who provides primary health care to women, particularly during birth but also across the lifespan. Usually linked by a shared philosophy of care, midwives may have nursing degrees and other advanced training in midwifery.

OR: Short for "operating room," where cesareans and other surgeries almost always take place.

pitocin: An intravenous medication often given to start or hasten labor or reduce bleeding after birth; a synthetic form of the naturally occurring hormone oxytocin.

placenta: A temporary organ that connects the fetus (through the umbilical cord) and the pregnant woman (through the wall of her uterus), and that serves as place where nutrients, oxygen, and waste are exchanged. The placenta is delivered after the child and is sometimes called the *afterbirth*.

previa: A condition in which the placenta is close to or covering the cervix. Previa may result in heavy bleeding before or during labor, and requires delivery by cesarean if it persists through pregnancy.

ultrasound: Refers in pregnancy to a test in which high-frequency sound waves are used to project an image of the fetus onto a screen; sometimes called a *sonogram*.

vacuum: A flexible rounded cup attached to a suction pump, sometimes placed on the baby's head to assist delivery.

VBAC: Short for *Vaginal Birth After Cesarean*; indicates a birth in which a woman has delivered a previous child by cesarean.

Index